Also by Michael F. Roizen and Mehmet C. Oz

YOU: The Owner's Manual

YOU: The Owner's Manual for Teens

YOU: On a Diet

YOU: Losing Weight

YOU: Staying Young

YOU: Being Beautiful

YOU: Having a Baby

YOU: Raising Your Child

YOU: Stress Less

YOU: On a Walk

YOU: The Smart Patient

YOU(r) TEEN: LOSING WEIGHT

The Owner's Manual to Simple and Healthy Weight Management at Any Age

MICHAEL F. ROIZEN, MD
ELLEN ROME, MD, MPH
MEHMET C. OZ, MD

with Ted Spiker, Craig Wynett, Zoe Oz,

Linda G. Kahn, MPH and Jeffrey D. Roizen, MD, PhD

FREE PRESS

New York   London   Toronto   Sydney   New Delhi

Free Press
A Division of Simon & Schuster, Inc.
1230 Avenue of the Americas
New York, NY 10020

First Free Press trade paperback edition January 2013

FREE PRESS and colophon are trademarks of Simon & Schuster, Inc.

For information about special discounts for bulk purchases, please contact Simon & Schuster Special Sales at 1-866-506-1949 or business@simonandschuster.com.

The Simon & Schuster Speakers Bureau can bring authors to your live event. For more information or to book an event contact the Simon & Schuster Speakers Bureau at 1-866-248-3049 or visit our website at www.simonspeakers.com.

Manufactured in the United States of America

1 3 5 7 9 10 8 6 4 2

ISBN 978-1-4767-1357-1

ISBN 978-1-4767-1358-8 (ebook)

To all those who think
regaining your life is hard—
we hope this makes it much easier.
You are worth it.

YOU(r) TEEN: LOSING WEIGHT

INTRODUCTION

Weight Management

Every stage of life has its share of obstacles. As a middle-aged adult, you may experience all kinds of life stress—from emotional to financial and everything in between. As an older adult, you may have a little more trouble walking or seeing or doing any number of things that you used to be able to do. As an infant, it would be nice if you could articulate (in a way other than wailing your brains out) that, yeah, you could use a diaper change right about now.

But of all the stages in life, many folks would argue that the teen years—with all of the ups, downs, and in-betweens of freaky and fiery hormones—can be, well, more complex than a rocket engine.

Of course, at this age there are plenty of joys and triumphs, and life is full of energy and possibilities. But it is also tricky to navigate the physical and emotional waters of school, of sports, of trying to fit in, of deciding between the blue or purple shirt, of wigging out about the fact that now is not exactly the best time for a nose zit to take center stage.

For many of us, it's hard to remember—and really appreciate—the angst that teenagers go through every day.

When you throw in an added element—that of being overweight or obese, which some 40 percent of teens in our country are—you've just swirled up that emotional concoction and put the blender on high.

That's what *YOU(r) Teen: Losing Weight* is all about: slowing down the blender and learning to put all the pieces together to help your teens live a healthy life.

We want to help. We want to give you a quick and simple-to-navigate guidebook that will teach you the ins and outs of fat, nutrition, exercise, emotions, and all of the important elements that go into a weight loss system. We know that this is a hard thing to talk about. You don't want to talk about weight, ask for help, or ask for tonight's dinner to be carrot burgers and spinach because that's what's most healthful.

But you do want to change.

And the great news—to contrast with many of the other challenges that teens have—is that if teens are able to make a change their bodies are more plastic (more responsive) to that change than your body may be.

So what our goal is here is to teach you not only what works in terms of weight loss but how to create an environment so that weight loss isn't a struggle but rather something that comes as naturally as that aforementioned pimple (but with more desired results). As a bonus, of course, many of these strategies are things that will work for anyone trying to lose weight, so it can also be used as a way to help the whole family change if need be.

In this book, we'll first take you through the biology of weight gain and loss, because we always feel that the "why" element is an important precursor to the "what." We don't especially think you need to dole out biology lessons across the dinner table every night ("Pass the broccoli, and let's activate some GLP-1!"), but we do believe that being armed with this information will give you teaching moments to discuss the body and how it works. After learning the biology, we'll give you the strategies and tips that you can employ to lose weight. At the back of the book, we'll provide some great recipes, a sample two-week diet plan, and three workouts that will help burn calories and build stronger bodies. Hey, maybe your teen will even let you work out with her.

There's little doubt that we're a country that has some tremendous health issues. We want to set you on the right track with behaviors that will help for a lifetime. We believe that dieting doesn't have to be hard (though we know that getting through to any teen can be more difficult than trying to hammer a nail with a banana) but rather has to be smart. And we hope that's what you will get out of this book—the knowledge that can make it easier to sustain your weight loss—and that can lead to motivation that can lead to action that helps you achieve and sustain the weight you want.

And that's what can lead to a healthy, happy life.

PART 1

Biology Lessons

Before any discussion about how hunger and exercise work, it's important to take a look at the offender that's at the center (quite literally) of this whole issue: fat.

Of course, for overweight folks, the extra fat is sure to manifest itself in some outward side effects, such as lack of energy or lack of self-esteem. But many of the risk factors associated with carrying too much fat don't have any outward symptoms at all—meaning that the only way to tell whether being overweight is threatening your life is by taking a microscope underneath the flub and chub and focusing on what's happening at your body's core levels. This is especially tricky for teens, who typically don't focus on the future but rather have the mentality "What have you done for me lately?" So they don't see the dangers lurking in their bodies. But they're real, and they need to be understood before starting any discussion.

The key anatomical player in all of this is an organ called the omentum. Why should we care about that organ that sounds as though it's missing the letter *m*? Because the omentum can store fat that is quickly accessible to the liver (meaning that it can cause "bad" cholesterol and triglyceride levels to rise), and it also sucks insulin out of circulation (preventing it from acting elsewhere and making your blood sugar rise)— meaning that the fat sets up shop in the omentum and puts your organs at risk of being damaged by that fat.

See, what's important about fat is like what's important about real estate: it's all about location, location, location.

We all have three kinds of fat: fat in our bloodstream (those are the triglycerides), subcutaneous fat (which lies just underneath the skin's surface), and that omental fat. (The fourth fat, of course, is the fat in food.) The omentum is a fatty layer of tissue located inside the belly behind the muscles in your abdomen (that's why some men with beer guts have a hard-as-keg outside to their bellies—their fat is underneath the outer muscle).

Because this omentum fat—the belly fat, if you will—is so close to your solid organs, it's their first and worst energy source. (Why go to the gas station on the other side of town when there's a station at the next corner?) Think of the omentum fat as an obnoxious eighteen-wheeler on a crowded highway—elbowing out the stomach, pushing other organs away, and claiming all the space for itself.

What's most interesting—and encouraging—is that as soon as you change your omentum, your body starts seeing effects. That is, once your body senses it's losing that fat, its blood-related numbers (cholesterol, blood pressure, blood sugar) start traveling in the healthy direction—within days, before you even notice any kind of physical sign of weight loss. Changing your omentum changes your metabolic momentum!

For your health, what you really want to do is get those blood numbers to be in a healthy range. By doing that, you'll lower your risk of heart disease, diabetes, high blood pressure, high cholesterol—and all of the things that serve as real health dangers.

And when your teen's body is in the right balance, you all benefit. He's in a better mood, has better energy and higher self-esteem, and is a happier person. Everyone wins.

And those are things that teens surely understand.

THE BIOLOGY OF HUNGER

To talk about weight and waist size, you have to talk about two key elements: portion size and food choices—yes, both matter big time. Eat too much, and you're going to be sporting extra pounds; eat too little, and you're going to screw up your metabolism. Either way, you alter your body's biological processes and set yourself up for some serious health problems.

Here we'd like to give you an overview of the basics of good nutrition—food choices that give you energy. You may know that foods are essentially broken into three subcategories: protein (found in meat, fish, eggs, nuts, and beans), carbohydrates (found in grains, fruits, and vegetables), and fats (found in butter, eggs, meat, fish, oils, and nuts). Each one serves different purposes in the body; protein, for example, is an essential building block of muscle. But they all serve one main purpose: providing energy to your bodily systems and organs.

All food is eventually broken down into units the body can use. Protein is broken down into amino acids, the foundation of every cell in your body. Fats are utilized to protect nerve cells and are an excellent source of energy that can be stored for long-term use. The sugars in carbohydrates are all converted to glucose, the body's principal source of energy. Many people think that the way you get fat is by eating fat. That can be true, but it's misleading. Any of the three types of nutrients can make you fat if you ingest too much of it. As your body processes food, it shuttles its nutrients throughout your body—to feed your brain or fuel your biceps. Any extras that can't be used are essentially put into a doggie bag and saved for later, in the form of fat stored in your body. Although the different kinds of nutrients can be interconverted, they have different effects on your feeling full and on your body's metabolism.

Healthful eating entails paying attention to both the quality and the quantity of food you consume. You want enough calories to keep your body energized, while at the same time making sure that your meals are balanced with foods from each of the three groups. Furthermore, you want to make sure you're choosing healthful options from within each food group. Think of the sugar rush you get when you drink a Coke and eat a sugary cereal for breakfast. Now compare that to the feeling you get when you eat a bowl of oatmeal with a glass of low-fat milk. They may contain the same number of calories, but one meal is packed with nutrients, while the other is made up mostly of sugar. The healthy choice—the oatmeal, in case you hadn't figured it out—contains fiber and a little bit of fat, which takes longer to digest, so you stay fuller longer. It also contains nutrients that improve your body's function and fight disease. The unhealthful choice might give you an initial burst of energy, but its calories are nutritionally "empty" and will only lead you to crash and crave another fix.

The quality and quantity of food you eat have a major influence on your appetite regulation—how your body and brain know they want or need more food. Let's take a look at how it all works.

In the center of your brain sits the hypothalamus, a key command center for your body. Among the biological functions it controls are temperature, metabolism, and sex drive. The tiny structure also controls your appetite—not just for food but also for thirst, sleep, and even for that special someone. Hidden in your hypothalamus is a satiety center that regulates your appetite for food by responding to two hormones that regulate whether you feel hungry or full: ghrelin and leptin.

Here's how they work. Your stomach and intestines do more than hold food and produce belches that register on the Richter scale. When your stomach is empty, its inner lining releases a feisty little chemical called ghrelin. When your stomach is growling, it's that gremlin of a hormone that's sending desperate messages that you need more food. Ghrelin makes you want to eat. When you diet by depriving yourself (not eating enough food), the increased ghrelin secretion sends even more signals to eat, overriding your willpower and causing chemical reactions that give you little choice but to go crazy in the pantry. Your stomach secretes ghrelin in pulses every half hour, sending subtle chemical impulses to your brain—almost like subliminal biological messages: Cheese fries! Milk shake! Triple burger! When you're *really* hungry, those messages come fast—every twenty minutes or so—and they're also amplified. So you get more and stronger signals that your body wants food. After a long period, your body often can't ignore those messages. The chemical cattle prod stops when you eat; when your stomach fills, your ghrelin levels go down, thus reducing your appetite. Even if you're not dieting, if you miss a meal (say, breakfast) this signal gets stronger.

On the other hand, there's leptin, produced mainly by fat tissue; it tells your brain that your body is full. Here's how the two work together: Ghrelin works in the short term, sending out those hunger signals two or three times an hour. Leptin works in the long term, so if you can get your leptin signals up, you'll have a greater ability to keep your appetite in check. Leptin can outrank ghrelin.

But all foods are not created equal when it comes to stimulating leptin. In particular, highly processed foods, especially those that contain high-fructose corn syrup (HFCS—recently rebranded as corn sugar), are less likely to stimulate leptin production or leptinlike response from your brain than foods containing a healthful balance of protein, fat, and carbohydrates.

The fructose in HFCS, which is used to sweeten soft drinks and salad dressings, among many other foods, isn't—in contrast to the type of fructose found in fruit—seen by your brain as a regular food, so it doesn't tell your body to stop eating. Even low-fat foods that contain HFCS can wind up high in calories, partly because you overeat without the brain signaling "Hey! You're full! Put down that fork!"

The power struggle between ghrelin and leptin also involves other chemicals, specifically those that influence mood, such as serotonin (more on that in a moment). Ever notice how easy it is to drown your sorrows in a pint of Häagen-Dazs? That's because simple sugars in foods such as ice cream increase your levels of this neurotransmitter, which makes you feel good. But that feeling quickly fades, and your brain, craving to feel good again, commands you to seek more of those simple sugars to recapture that feeling. And when you don't get enough sleep, your ghrelin level goes up and your leptin level goes down; it's why we crave sweet and starchy foods when we're tired, to give us that pick-me-up feeling.

The bottom line is that by eating healthful foods and limiting unhealthful foods—the five food felons, below—you actually nudge your hormones to work in your favor and essentially outmuscle hormonal urges to overeat. In our tips section, you'll find plenty of tips that will help do just that.

THE BIOLOGY OF MOVEMENT

A word that a lot of people like to throw around like a Frisbee at a picnic: metabolism. His is fast, mine is slow. But what is it? And how does it work? Of course, most of us equate metabolism with either genetics or exercise. Both are right, but let's take a look at what metabolism means and why exercise is so important.

By definition, metabolism is the rate at which you burn

the calories you consume. But get this—only 15 to 30 percent of your daily intake of calories is burned through intentional physical activity such as exercise, walking, or dancing.

Your body burns most of the calories you consume by keeping the heart pumping, the brain remembering math equations—just performing everyday functions. However, that doesn't mean that outside influences don't slow down and speed up your burn rate. Any movement speeds metabolism, including fidgeting (called "nonexercise activity thermogenesis" in scientific lingo, or NEAT for short). Every increase in body temperature of 1 degree increases your metabolic rate by 14 percent. Eating protein appears to do the same thing naturally, by the way. When you sleep, your metabolic rate decreases by 10 percent. Perhaps most shockingly, when you starve yourself for more than twelve hours, your metabolic rate actually goes down by 40 percent. This is because when you skip meals, your body senses a dietary disaster (it thinks, "Oh, no, a famine!") and quickly goes into storage mode rather than burning mode. That's how our ancestors survived famines: by storing fat when they were deprived of food. There you have the primary reason why deprivation diets don't work for losing weight. It's also why skipping breakfast ruins your day; you have less energy because your body is saving up for the famine.

Some of your metabolism is genetic; you're born with a certain burn rate. That's why some rail-thin people can eat a lot and not get fat (which doesn't necessarily mean they're healthy, by the way). But you can control your metabolism to some extent by eating steadily throughout the day rather than bingeing and by consuming good-for-you foods (or at least by not missing meals). One of the ways you can really influence your metabolic rate is through exercise. Even though it makes up only a portion of the metabolic equation, it is one you can control.

Of course, there's no doubt that exercise has many benefits:

❑ It increases your metabolism so that you burn energy at a faster rate than if you don't exercise.

❑ It increases your brain size, which increases your metabolic rate the most (your brain uses the most energy of any of your organs).

❑ It reduces your appetite.

❑ It helps you sleep better.

❑ It stimulates the release of endorphins, chemicals that stimulate the pleasure centers in the brain.

❑ It helps decrease depression and increase positive attitude.

❑ It decreases the risk of lots of health problems, such as heart trouble and even memory problems.

The two most important components, when it comes to movement, are your muscles and your heart.

Muscles. We have almost 650 of them in our bodies, and they all play a part in helping to give us the strength not only to perform well in sports but also to get our bodies through the day.

Muscles are made up of tissues that contract and relax. They're kind of like an extendable ladder that snaps together and shortens when you pull or apply tension at one end.

When you release the tension on the muscle or ladder, it relaxes and extends. Your energy intake (healthful food, not flaming nacho cheesy fries) provides the power for your muscles to contract and relax. Work them and feed them right, and they will grow. Starve yourself long enough, and you'll start breaking them down to fuel the rest of your body and little by little get weaker. Eventually you'll start to notice it, unless all your attention is elsewhere, as happens with eating disorders. In fact, when your body thinks you are starving (or in a famine because you skipped breakfast), you break down muscle before you break down fat.

Muscles grow after they're used. Lifting weights, doing push-ups, or performing any other kind of exercise that requires you to push or pull damages the muscle fibers; the soreness you may feel afterward comes from the toxins released by muscle tissue when it is damaged. When you're done, the muscles say, "Forget this, we're not going to be damaged again. We're going to build up to be even stronger than before," which is why they get larger. For those who are overweight or looking to maintain weight loss, the great thing is that muscle actually helps you burn fat much faster than fat or other tissue. So if you're looking to lose weight, in addition to watching your calorie intake, build some muscle to increase the fat-burning engines in your body.

Heart. You may think about the heart when it comes to other things in life—relationships, for instance—but that blood pumper plays the starring role when it comes to exercise. As your body moves and burns fuel in the form of the sugar called glucose to produce energy, it requires oxygen, and your heart has to beat faster to circulate more oxygen-rich blood to the tissues that need it. (The motion is less like the beating drum that we typically think of; it's more like the wringing out of a wet towel. The heart squeezes blood to pump it in and out of the circulatory system.) At the same time, your blood picks up waste in the form of carbon dioxide and carries it back to your lungs, where it is breathed out and fresh oxygen is breathed in.

Some people think the heart is the most important part of the body, as reflected in phrases such as "the heart of the matter." That may very well be true, but raising your heart rate—through exercises such as running, swimming, cycling, playing basketball, and many other activities—also helps increase metabolism and burn fat.

Ideally, what we're after is engaging in movement and exercise that works both systems—the muscles as well as the cardiovascular system. There are all kinds of strategies to use to get them moving, especially if your primary movement system involves thumbs, and we'll go over them in part 2.

THE BIOLOGY OF EMOTIONS

As you well know, emotional eating isn't about reaching for celery. Rather, it's out-of-control, often bingey, hedonistic eating, where you eat every cookie in the bag because they look good and taste even better. It's a craving—and usually for something that's starchy, sugary, salty, or loaded with fat.

For teens, emotional eating may come in different forms. They may eat because they're depressed or stressed or in a bad mood or just plain bored.

The following five brain chemicals are the ones that primarily influence our emotions; not only do they provide the foundation for why we eat at certain times, but they're also the key chemicals altered by many of our current and future weight loss drugs—because they tend to regulate some of the reasons *why* we eat certain foods (and certain amounts of foods).

Norepinephrine and cortisol. These caveman, fight-or-flight hormones tell you to tangle with a saber-toothed tiger or hightail it to the safety of your hut.

Serotonin. It's a neurotransmitter that makes you feel good and is a major target of antidepression drugs.

Dopamine. It's the brain's fun house. It's a pleasure-and-reward system and is particularly sensitive to addictions. It's also the one that helps you feel no pain.

GABA (gamma-aminobutyric acid). This amino acid makes you feel like a zombie and is one of the ways that anesthesia may work to reduce your responsiveness to the outside world.

Nitric oxide. This meditation-like chemical helps calm you. This powerful neuropeptide is usually very short lived gas; it also relaxes the blood vessels of the body.

Now, the real question is: what do all these chemicals have to do with whether or not you snack on a Hershey bar or a plum? Probably the best way to think about it is to use serotonin as an example. Picture your brain as a small pinball machine. You have millions of neurotransmitters that are sending messages to and from one another. When your serotonin transmitters fire the signals (from the flippers), they send the message throughout your brain that you feel good; this message is strongest when that feel-good pinball is frenetically bouncing around in your brain, racking up tons of yeah-baby points along the way. But when you lose the ball down the chute (that is, when cells in the brain take the serotonin and break it down), that love-the-world feeling you've just been experiencing is lost. So what does your brain want to do? Put another quarter in the machine and get another ball. For many of us, the next ball comes in the form of foods that usually (and quickly) make us feel good, to counteract the drop in serotonin that we're feeling.

Unfortunately, the way we typically satisfy our urge to play another ball is to consume foods that provide an immediate rush of serotonin. That rush can come with a jolt of sugar, which stimulates the release of serotonin. Insulin facilitates serotonin production in the brain, which in turn boosts our mood, makes us feel better, or masks the stress, pain, boredom, anger, or frustration that we may be feeling. But serotonin is only one ball in play. You have all sorts of other chemicals fighting to send your appetite and cravings from bumper to bumper.

To see how the total picture works, think of these chemicals as parts of a scale. When the chemicals associated with positive feelings (such as serotonin and dopamine) are in the up (or activated) position, you're chemically high. But when they're down, you experience a big emotional and chemical downfall. That puts you into a state of anxiety that sends you searching for the foods, especially simple carbohydrates, that will get you back to the chemical high. That's how illegal drugs work too; users keep seeking the high not always for its own sake but to avoid the lows. It's a constant fight to get back to that place of neurochemical comfort.

When these chemicals are high, your weight gets lower, and when they're lower, you reach for the foods that will eventually make your weight higher. That's the reason why what happens inside your skull plays such a vital role in what happens under your belt.

So what's the goal? To keep the feel-good hormones level so there's a steady state of satisfaction with no huge hormonal highs and lows that make you search for good-for-your-brain-but-bad-for-your-waistline foods.

The reality is that a good number of teens with weight problems have emotional issues that run deeper than the middle of the Pacific and try to satisfy their need for fulfillment by self-medicating with food.

For some people, being overweight is really about lack of self-esteem—about the petrifying fear that they don't deserve to be thin. How do we know this? Not through studies or research but through real-life living, through our patients, through eavesdropping on a cavalcade of doughnut addicts.

18

Here, we have to momentarily step out of the safety zone of hard science into an area that's typically not studied by the white-coat-and-goggles set, because the mental, emotional, and deep psychological issues involved with obesity are simply very difficult to "prove" in a Western sense.

So let's start here. Many people lack the self-esteem for waist control. But let's dive deeper: what is self-esteem? Let's assume that our general sense of self-worth comes from two forces: overcoming obstacles and accomplishing some kind of goal. In the case of waist management, what happens if you don't overcome a challenge (avoiding a box of Ding Dongs) and don't accomplish something (reaching your goal weight by the end of summer)?

Yep, your self-esteem plummets faster than the ratings of summer reruns. To resurrect it, you need to find ways to overcome the challenges and accomplish the goals—without making the standards by which you measure your life unrealistic weights, measurements, and stricter-than-boot-camp eating habits.

There are some chemical and biological foundations for the feeling of soul-level satisfaction that comes with finding your own special "it"—whatever that "it" may be (it's different for everyone). One theory is that oxytocin (a hormone that is elevated in women after childbirth, by the way) makes you feel a sense of community and pleasure when you are within your family, are satisfied with a loved one or friend, have a religious experience, or have an epiphany about your existence. When your oxytocin levels increase, you feel calm. Another hypothesis argues that your sense of self-esteem and well-being is influenced by the chemical nitric oxide (not to be confused with laughing gas, nitrous oxide). Traits such as hopefulness and optimism are associated with the release of nitric oxide through the body. In the same way, the release of nitric oxide may serve to help reduce feelings of anxiety and stress. But this chemical effect lasts for only seconds, so you need to continually stimulate your body with the right cerebral karma (hope and optimism).

Whether it's the result of oxytocin, nitric oxide, or both, soul-level satisfaction exists at a biochemical level as well as in your perceptible life. It's your deeper drive—not the drive to fill the needs of your stomach or your muscles or even your mind but the drive to fill the needs of your soul.

Okay, okay, okay, we know what you're saying: what does your soul have to do with the fact that you just mainlined an entire bag of chips?

A lot. Many of us, instead of addressing—or even acknowledging—this deeper longing and the restlessness we feel for never quite fulfilling it try to fill the emptiness with food and drink. We use a temporary fix (leftover pizza for breakfast) to satisfy not only the chemical cravings but also the permanent void caused by not satisfying our spiritual needs (the "it").

Of all the actions you pursue, one of the few things you totally control is eating. You have the freedom to chow down on what you want, where you want, and how you want, and whether you want to do it with or without clothes on. This freedom is particularly appealing to those in our culture, such as teenagers, who may feel that they lack choices or freedom. They hunger for love, they hunger for power, they hunger for respect, and they hunger for meaning, but all of those things may be out of their control, or seem to be. They hunger for nachos—and bam! that they can control. Because of that freedom and choice, eating makes you feel good. Funny thing, though; food is like the paint you use to cover cracks in the foundation of your house. Two coats of robin's-egg blue may hide the flaws temporarily, but they're never going to fix the real root of the problem. If this is you, your cover-up (emotional eating) is what starts that tornadolike cycle that keeps you from ever feeling satisfied physically or emotionally.

So part of a strong weight loss plan is to find your passion. Discover what motivates you, what jazzes you, what makes you happy—a place where you can exert control, can gain expertise (and perhaps some sense of power, respect, and meaning) through application of hard work. Because with that foundation, the other elements of weight loss more easily fall into place.

THE BIOLOGY: PUTTING IT ALL TOGETHER

If you take the definition of a perfect storm, you'll realize that it's not just a bunch of bad stuff that happens all at once. Rather, it is a concurrence of events that, taken individually, are relatively insignificant but when combined can have powerful consequences. That's absolutely the case when it comes to fat. Just look at all the factors that contribute to our growing size: biological, environmental, political, emotional, and so on. No matter what their origin, there are a lot of them. Consider these individual reasons:

- ❏ We're hardwired to want sugar, salt, and fat. And they're readily available in every fast-food joint and packaged food, even if you don't realize it.
- ❏ Your body stores fat to protect against famine.
- ❏ Your moods and social situations can dictate cravings. You feast on cream-filled goodies when you're stressed. When the family gets together on Sunday, it's a calzone feast.
- ❏ Junk-food ads are all over the place. Biological forces called mirror neurons make us crave what we see, and the marketing machine pushes all the right buttons.
- ❏ The mass production of high-fructose corn syrup has made it easier to gobble down pounds and pounds of sugar every year in the plethora of processed foods that we eat.
- ❏ We sit more than ever (blame desk jobs for adults, video games for kids, and TV for both).
- ❏ There are fast-food joints and convenience stores at every corner. One study even found that high schoolers whose school is within a quarter mile of fast-food places have a BMI higher than those who aren't as close.
- ❏ Schools and offices are littered with vending machines filled with foods that have empty carbohydrates.
- ❏ Kids don't walk to school as they used to a few decades ago, and forty thousand elementary schools have eliminated recess from the school day, decreasing children's total time of activity.
- ❏ We've become a car culture; housing developments are often far from shops, and many neighborhoods don't even have sidewalks.

We—and we're sure you—could go on and on with other reasons as well. Each factor by itself is no big deal. Put them all together, and this button-popping storm can destroy every organ in its path.

Why do we tell you this? Our point is that we know darn well how hard it is to lose weight, maintain a healthy weight and waist size, and confront all of life's challenges. We also know that it's impossible to outbrute, outpunch, and outwill those forces.

Anybody who remembers the movie *The Perfect Storm* and the powerful wave that doomed the ship knows that you can't fight a perfect storm; you can't outslug it, and you can't stand stoically in the face of it. Instead, you have to get out of that evil sucker. Even a powerful ship can get clobbered in a perfect storm no matter what measures it takes.

But if you know the factors contributing to the storm and can track the storm to avoid it in the first place, you can beat it.

That's the whole point: to ride out a perfect storm, you have to change your environment from stormy seas to calm ones.

That's really what this whole issue is about: changing your environment to change your behavior.

Face it, we need to eat every few hours, and we do have dopamine receptors that cause us to crave certain foods, such as sweets. So what should we do? Don't fight your biology; rather, change the environment to make your biology work for you, not against you. In practical terms, that means you need to change your environment so you're less likely to be caught in a storm. Keep fruit in your kitchen instead of chips.

And when you eat out? Choose a fish (nonfried, as of now[*]) place rather than a burger joint. While there's nothing earth-shattering about snacking on fruit or ordering a lean piece of fish, the Aha! moment comes when you learn not to fight the wave—by denying yourself the pleasure of dining out, for example—but to ride the wave by adjusting the environment to your behaviors.

Fundamentally, you want to make it easier to do the right thing.

Choose what you or those you shop for are going to eat while you are in the supermarket—actually, before you go to the supermarket (make a list in advance, and stick to it)—rather than when the fridge door is off its hinges as you scavenge for food. By planning ahead, instead of scooping up leftover cheesecake you'll find a bunch of fresh grapes.

What you'll see is that environment can influence biology. You don't need to employ DEFCON 5 willpower against a candy bar if there are no candy bars in the house. You will reach for carrot sticks if that's what's around.

Environment is everything in the weight loss battle, and as a parent, you have the power (and maybe responsibility?) to create an environment that gives you the best shot at your best health.

---

[*] Researchers are working on a fryer that will use some new oils that will make fried food "health food"—but they aren't there yet (and may never get there).

PART 2

Your Strategies

Now that you've learned the why, it's time to learn the how, as in how to do it. We believe that understanding biology will help give you the knowledge and motivation to make meaningful changes, so we hope our biology lesson was useful. That said, just knowing the why doesn't get things done. The why doesn't tell you what foods to avoid and strategies to use when you're face to face with foods that are more evil than an *Avengers* villain. This part of the book will give you the foundation to help you make healthy living easy (and fun). You can find many more tips and tricks in *YOU on a Diet*, revised and updated.

Know good versus not good. Generally, ingredients can be classified into these two groups. By knowing which foods fall into which categories, you'll go a long way toward making lasting changes—and making smart choices at every meal and snack.

> *Healthful ingredients:* lean protein (such as skinless turkey and chicken, fish), healthful fats (such as omega-3 fatty acids, unsaturated fats), healthful carbohydrates (100 percent whole grain), fiber (oatmeal, vegetables, psyllium husks).

Unhealthful ingredients: the five food felons: (1) added simple sugars, (2) enriched (or bleached or refined) flour, (3) added syrups such as HFCS (also called corn sugar), (4) saturated fats (four-legged animal fat, two-legged animal skin, coconut and palm oils), and (5) trans fats.

First, avoid simple sugars and syrups. Saturated fats and trans fats are other ingredients to avoid. Finally, stay clear of enriched, bleached, and refined flour. All three words mean that the flour has been stripped of its nutrients. All of these in excess can contribute to obesity and lead to other long-term health risks. Use flour made 100 percent with whole grains instead.

The ideal is to eat these healthful foods in balance: a little protein, healthful fats, and healthful carbs at each of your meals. Lean proteins include chicken, turkey, fish (great for those omega-3 fatty acids). Healthful fats (you need at least 30 to 50 grams worth a day) include olives, natural peanut butter, olive oil, hummus, and many other Mediterranean-style foods. Healthful carbs that can also give you needed fiber include things cooked with chia seeds and whole grain flour, anything whole grain, whole wheat pasta, brown rice, and don't forget your fruits and veggies.

Don't undereat. When our ancestors couldn't find food and went for long periods of time without it, their bodies acted like life preservers, storing fat in anticipation of the inevitable periods of famine. The same system works today. When you try to "diet" by going for long periods of time without eating or by eating way too few calories, your brain senses the starvation and sends an SOS signal through your body to store fat because famine is on its way. That's why people who go on extreme fasts and extremely low-calorie diets don't lose the expected weight. They store fat as a natural protective mechanism. To lose weight, you have to keep your body from switching into starvation mode. The only way to do it: eat often, in the form of frequent healthful meals and snacks.

Ballpark (don't obsess) the calories. Some people like to count calories; others can't stand it. So if you are tech-minded, you may like to do the math and track calories. But it's not necessary, especially since there's such a wide range of caloric requirements depending on individual needs. Most teens need a minimum of 2,000 calories a day just to keep their bodies functioning. But athletes—and those of us growing (most teens are!)—may need significantly more than that. Those who are actively trying to lose weight shouldn't go below 1,500 to 1,800 calories a day.

Automate your eating. If any waist management plan is going to work—as in *really* work—eating right has to become as automatic as it was for our ancestors. That's not as insurmountable as it seems. Just look at one study from *The Journal of the American Medical Association.* Two groups were assigned two different diets. One went on a diet rich in good-for-YOU foods such as whole grains, fruits, vegetables, nuts, and olive oil, foods found in the typical Mediterranean diet. The other group was not given any specific direction in terms of foods to eat but was instructed to consume specific percentages of fat, carbohydrates, and protein daily. In short, they had to think a lot about preparing foods and dividing amounts, while the first group had only general guidelines about foods to eat. The groups weren't given guidelines about how much to eat; they let their hunger levels dictate their hunger patterns. When they did that, what happened? Without trying, the first group consumed fewer calories, lost inches, and dropped pounds. The point: the people in the "good-for-YOU-foods group" ate the foods that naturally kept them satiated so that their bodies could seek their playing weights.

- ❏ The "good-for-YOU-foods group" consumed significantly more fiber than the control group.
- ❏ The "good-for-YOU-foods group" consumed higher amounts of good-for-YOU omega-3 and omega-9 fats in the form of olives, fish, and nuts (especially walnuts). Those fats help increase the level of chemicals that make you feel satiated.
- ❏ The "good-for-YOU-foods group" more than doubled their consumption of fruits and vegetables.
- ❏ The "good-for-YOU-foods group" ate the foods we recommend here, didn't obsess about calories, and enabled their bodies to do what they're supposed to do: regulate the chemicals that are responsible for hunger and for satiety.

Pick and stick. Yeah, sure, variety may be the spice of life, but it can also be the death of healthful eating. When you have lots of choices for a meal, it's much easier to slip out of good eating habits and into fried-ham-induced bad ones. One way to avoid excess fat intake is to eliminate choices for at least one meal a day. For teens, that's most often breakfast. So find two or three healthful breakfasts that you like—say, oatmeal, cereal with low-fat milk, yogurt with fruit, or all-natural peanut butter on 100 percent whole wheat bread—and stick to them every day. Every day. Yes, every day. When you make it an automatic choice, you won't make errors by choosing something unhealthful.

Expand your horizons. Here's a concept we're betting you've never heard quite this way: obesity is an infectious disease. No, it's not as if anyone's going to sneeze cheeseburger bits into your arteries. Nevertheless, there is a major infectious component to obesity; it spreads through social networks. Just consider one study that shows that if one of two friends is obese, the other's chance of becoming obese increases by 171 percent. That's why it's crucial to consider what and *whom* you surround yourself with. If you socialize with the everyday-is-a-reason-to-eat-lasagna crowd, chances are that you're going to be knee deep in ricotta without much chance of digging out (except with a fork). But if you're surrounded by a set of healthy friends, you'll adopt more healthful habits. Does that mean we suggest that you ditch any overweight friends? Of course not. But maybe it means that you should get out more with friends who have more healthful habits. Let their good habits rub off on you.

Don't fret the fat. A lot of people, especially teens, think that eating fat means they'll get fat. That's not quite right. Consuming too many calories—whether in the form of protein, carbohydrates, or fat—is what contributes to weight gain. But as discussed, the key to controlling weight gain is to eat the right foods that will help keep your appetite hormones level so you don't get those intense hunger pangs that make you feel like gorging. Your brain actually needs healthful fat in your diet. Fat in your brain is not excess-calorie fat; it's used to myelinate (or hard wire) your neural pathways, helping you learn or become more coordinated. Without adequate fat, your brain capacity shrinks. DHA omega-3 fat makes up about 60 percent of the fat in your brain. It is your "smart fat."

Here's a little more about fat. Many teens and adults aim for a low-fat diet in an attempt to be healthy. What many don't realize is that a low-fat diet does not mean a *no-fat* diet. Your brain and body need a minimum of 30 to 50 grams of healthful fat a day for a reasonable-fat diet, and a standard diet can easily include 70 to 90 grams of fat a day. Many dieters think that it's okay to eat only 5 to 15 grams a day, to eat no items that have 5 to 8 grams of fat in them, or to obey other extreme dieting dictates. Unfortunately, this is not the best strategy; lack of fat in a diet can lead to loss of myelin, the fatty sheaths that surround nerves and allow messages to be transmitted from brain to body and back. Moreover, the cerebral cortex—the part of the brain that does all of your key thinking—actually shrinks if you don't get enough dietary fat (and cardio-boosting activity) over a long enough period of time.

And if you need a selling point: besides keeping your brain fit and functioning, fat is responsible for the shine and texture of your hair and the firmness of breasts in girls; if you lose enough weight and body fat, the breasts get saggy. Healthful fats include olive oil and omega-3 fats from fish (especially salmon and trout), algae, walnuts, and avocados.

Plan your meals. Start every day knowing when and what you are going to eat. That way, you'll avert the 180-degree shift between starving and gorging that occurs when you skip meals. Almost one-third of U.S. youngsters eat fast food every day, meaning that they consume more calories and eat fewer good foods than on days when they don't eat fast food. Almost all schools offer healthful alternatives for lunch. If yours does not, why not pack a peanut butter sandwich on 100 percent whole wheat bread and a cut-up apple sprinkled with lemon juice? Or a chia meatball sandwich on 100 percent whole wheat bread (see page 61), a piece of fruit, a small bag of carrots for the crunch, and a water bottle.

Here's a waist management fact: bad foods aren't bad just because of the ingredients they contain but also because many of them are fast and easy, which are the exact traits that can get you into a whole lot of trouble—because you can consume many of them before you've even realized you've started. The key to successful dietary contingency plans is to have premade foods ready for those times when you've been conditioned to reach for bags of sugar-containing waistline killers. Instead, choose your favorites among these options to make once a week so you will have something to grab when you need it.

Cut-up vegetables. Your choice. Cut them, bag them, eat them. Nothing wrong with baby carrots, grape tomatoes, and broccoli florets, but if you prefer jicama, sugar snaps, and orange pepper strips, go for them.

Sautéed vegetables. Your choice. Sauté them in olive oil with chopped garlic, red pepper flakes, or a good dash of turmeric. Refrigerate and use for side dishes or hot (microwaved) snacks.

Soups. Make a filling soup once a week and store it in serving-size cups in the refrigerator (see our recipe for a good one). Eat 1 cup as a predinner appetizer to take the edge off your appetite, or have a cup of soup as a snack.

Steel-cut oats. If you're worried about time, cook up a week's worth of oats per directions and store in the refrigerator for up to a week. For some people, that might seem as appetizing as a slice of baked wrapping paper, but reheated oats actually taste great.

Emergency foods. Every house needs fire-extinguisher foods—good-for-you foods that will put out three-alarm starvation fires. Our list of foods that you can reach for when you're hungry include any of the above foods as well as a handful of almonds, peanuts, or walnuts; bags of store-bought, pre-chopped fruits and veggies; dried fruit (apricots, cranberries); and edamame (soybeans—look for microwave bags in the frozen food section). Avoid foods with added sugars. In a real pinch? Pop one of those mint breath strips—they can help turn off appetite by making food less appetizing.

Don't confuse thirst with hunger. The reason some people eat is that their satiety center is begging for attention. But sometimes, that appetite center wants things to quench thirst, not to fill the stomach. Thirst can be caused by hormones in the gut, or it can be a chemical response to eating; eating food increases the thickness of your blood, and your body senses the need to dilute it. A great way to counteract your hormonal reaction to food is to make sure that your response to thirst activation doesn't contain unnecessary, empty calories—like the ones in soft drinks and some juices. Your thirst center doesn't care whether it's getting zero-calorie water or a megacalorie frappe. When you feel hungry, drink a glass or two of water first to see if that's what your body really wants.

Think in terms of a weight range, not a set number. In all likelihood, the most common way you've measured your so-called dietary success or failure is by pounds lost. If you're down to your target weight, you've won. If not, you've lost. The reality is that over the long term, all of us intermittently gain and lose small amounts of weight, even when we're trying to lose it. For one, our water weight fluctuates depending on what we're eating. The reason that so many low-carb dieters lose weight fast is that the lack of carbohydrates causes them to lose glycogen stores from their muscles, and with that loss of glycogen comes a loss of a lot of water; as soon as they reinstate the carbs, the glycogen comes back into the muscles and attracts the water, which adds the pounds right back. So the first 5 to 11 pounds of weight loss on a low-carb diet is a fake loss due to a temporary loss of water. Instead of tracking your weight by a single goal weight of, say, 145 pounds, what you want to do is pick your weight class. Pick a range of weight that's comfortable for you—say, 142 to 148 pounds (or 31 to 33 inches of waist size). When you divulge your weight to someone (not that anyone will be asking), it should never be in terms of one number; you need to think of your weight as an ideal range. For one thing, it allows for the natural fluctuations that occur. For another, it does something even more crucial to your psychological success: it stops you from focusing on some arbitrary number that promotes the idea of all-or-nothing success or failure. And it puts your mind into the right programming mode—to remind yourself that your body is supposed to change. Also, after losing 10 percent of your weight, you may find it hard to lose more. The mechanisms your body uses to defend your weight redouble at that point. So you may want to aim for 9 percent weight loss and then maintenance for a while. Then repeat!

Get started exercising. If you haven't done any exercise, we recommend starting by simply walking thirty minutes a day at a brisk pace. (Wear running or walking shoes to provide the best support.) That will help you prepare a base level of fitness for your muscles and heart. We also recommend that you do our workout on page 64 that will challenge your muscles and make you stronger. Do it three times a week. You can complete it in 15 minutes, and it doesn't require any equipment. You don't even have to do formal exercise to get the benefits. Find something that makes your workout feel more like playing, and you'll still build your heart, muscles, and bones. It could be hiking or dancing or anything that gets your heart rate really going. Tennis is a game that you can learn now and play for life. Going for a walk in the woods once a month is lovely, but it doesn't count as regular exercise; you need to find something vigorous that you can do at least three times a week.

Know your fantastic four. Physical activity and exercise are like vegetables; they come in all shapes, sizes, and tastes, and just about all of them are good for you. Depending on your health level and experience, you need to be thinking about including these components of activity in your life:

Walking. We do it at the mall, around the house, and back and forth from the fridge to the bedroom. And, yes, any walking is healthful (the optimum is to hit at least 10,000 steps a day). But you also need to dedicate a total of 30 minutes a day to walking (broken up into chunks of at least 10 continuous minutes if you need to). It's the foundation for all other exercise because it not only increases your stamina but prepares your body for strength training. As a daily routine, walking is the psychological discipline that helps you stick with an activity plan. In fact, it has the highest compliance rate of any exercise. Commit to walking, and you'll start committing to more than just the TV lineup on Thursday nights.

Strength training. Even if the only barbell you've seen is the one that's piercing your buddy's tongue, that doesn't mean you should shy away from resistance training. Strength training—whether you use dumbbells, machines, bands, or your own body weight—helps rebuild muscle fibers and increase muscle mass, which will use up all those extra calories that you crave, so you can burn calories more efficiently and help prevent age-related weight gain. Here's the key to making it work. Many Americans spend a lot of time working their peripheral muscles (such as their biceps or their calves), but efficient strength training comes when you work the big muscles that make up the core axis of your body—your legs, the large muscles of your upper body (in your chest, shoulders, and back), your lower back muscles, and your abdominals. They're your foundation muscles. Best of all, you don't need a single piece of equipment to see the benefits. One quick note about abdominal exercises: they won't burn fat per se, but they will strengthen your entire core to help flatten and tone your stomach when you do burn fat. And they'll give you a layer of muscular support that will protect your lower back from injury. The tighter your abs, the less excess strain you'll cause your lower back. You can't build a house from the second floor down, and in a way your abdominal muscles and your entire core provide a base foundation that you can build upon.

Cardiovascular exercise. By doing cardiovascular exercise—that is, any activity that raises your heart rate for a sustained period of time—you'll increase your overall stamina, burn calories, and improve the function and efficiency of your heart, as well as lower your blood pressure. Sweating helps you to release toxins that would otherwise build up in your tissues.

Flexibility exercise. Being flexible isn't just a good trait for yoga teachers and potential spouses; it's also what you want for your muscles. Good flexibility helps prevent injuries to your joints, because stretching works your muscles through a wide range of motion that you'll go through during exercise and everyday activity. Being flexible makes you feel better; it keeps your body from feeling stiffer than a week-old roach corpse, helps facilitate meditation, and allows you to center yourself as you focus on your body. Plus, the more pliable and loose you are, the less you're affected when you fall or get into accidents.

Know these beginner guidelines. We don't want novices to overdo it right from the start (your best intentions can backfire if you start out too quickly), so keep these things in mind:

❏ Stay hydrated during exercise. That means guzzle water. You don't need energy drinks, which tend to contain lots of calories, unless you're exercising for more than an hour at full tilt or your doctor specifically tells you that you need the extra energy intake or need to gain weight. They rehydrate your body faster than plain water after long periods of exercise because they contain minerals and electrolytes that hasten the absorption of water. But if you drink nondiet sports drinks regularly, after short or not particularly strenuous workouts, or as pick-me-ups in the morning or afternoon, you'll end up consuming more calories than you burn. Also, avoid the ones with caffeine, as they can make you pee more, leaving you dehydrated.

❏ Remember that technique and good form are more important than how much weight you lift. You'll get stronger and reduce your risk of injury by doing exercise the right way. Before starting a weight-training regime, ask an instructor or trainer to show you the proper form.

❏ Don't think that exercise has to be boring or has to be done in gym class. Take a bike ride. Go for a hike. Use the stairs instead of the elevator. Find a workout buddy. You can always make smart choices about how to be more active in your everyday life.

❏ If you try to make dramatic changes all at once, you will set yourself up for failure. And if you try to binge diet or binge exercise, you will fail. When people try to make up for Thanksgiving sins at the table by going to the gym, the average person works off less than a third of the calories they have consumed. But a 20-minute walk each day combined with the gradual movement to the Mediterranean diet will make you thinner—at one month, at six months, and at ten years (and a great amount at each time).

❑ If you do fail for a meal by eating a bad burger or by forgetting to walk, the gradual and persistent changes you make will make it OK (as long as the trend is toward healthier meals and exercising most days each week).

Plan to fail—and develop contingency plans for when you do. We keep a tire in our trunk in case one goes flat. We keep candles in our drawers in case the power goes out. We keep backups of files in case our computers crash. (Some of us wish we backed them up more often.) That's good; contingency plans give you the mental assurance that you'll be able to adapt to unexpected crises. The one area where we don't make backup plans is in our diets. We eat broccoli, fish, and fruit for three days, then splurge on a double-fat burger with supersize fries on the fourth. For many of us, that's grounds for euthanizing the diet right away— putting us right back in touch with our three favorite food groups: chocolate, chips, and chocolate chips. Instead, start carrying a dietary contingency plan—a diet emergency pack for those times when you may experience a crash-causing blowout in one of your meals. That may mean taking a quick walk, doing a 10-minute workout, or just eating a handful of vegetables— something that will quickly recharge and refocus you.

THE DOWN LOW ON EATING DISORDERS

Living in the world today, many teens (and children and adults) are pretty conscious of their appearance in general and their weight and body shape in particular. It's nearly impossible to avoid the perfect-body-focused impact of society and the media. In addition, some people have individual and family factors that make them more susceptible to critical self-judgment and more demanding of personal "perfection." What's more, certain times and situations in life contribute huge amounts of stress and challenges. When all these factors combine in certain ways, it can create a setting for developing an eating disorder.

Eating disorders in their extreme form seem to burrow into the brains of their victims, taking over their thoughts and growing stronger every day. People with eating disorders build a "fat box," where every comment, every situation, is filtered through the box and distorted, so that it comes out as a criticism or demand. "You look great today" becomes "You usually look fat." "You look so healthy" becomes "You're eating too much." "I love your hair" becomes "I can't find anything nice to say about the rest of you."

Eating disorders also take over their victims' self-perceptions. People become unable to see the "real" image of themselves in the mirror, instead seeing someone much larger or with a distorted body shape. People with severe eating disorders often go to sleep thinking about food and wake up thinking about food. Every bite is an internal struggle. The "eating disorder voice" grows to be much louder than the individual's true voice, constantly berating and threatening: "You are a fat pig with no control!" "If you eat that cookie, you're going to be totally disgusting!"

A major part of fighting back against an eating disorder is for the sufferer to learn to hear and strengthen his or her own voice, so that he or she can make active decisions instead of giving power to the disorder. Though, to the outside observer, eating disorders seem to be all about the affected person's *behavior* related to food, they really are brain diseases, controlled by distortions in *thoughts* and *perceptions*. (Note: in milder forms, some bites or meals are challenges, but the thought process does not go on all the time.)

Eating disorders are another way to use food to try to exert control. People with anorexia nervosa (AN) have an intense fear of becoming fat or gaining any weight, even though they are often underweight. They seriously restrict their caloric intake and are generally acutely aware of every calorie that goes into their bodies. Besides restricting their food intake, people with anorexia may binge and purge, but the calories consumed are less than the average person consumes and much less than is needed for healthy functioning. People with bulimia nervosa (BN) have episodes of eating much more than the average person would eat in a particular time period, and they feel out of control of their eating during that time. Then they do something to "get rid of" the calories. This may include vomiting, using laxatives or other medications, fasting, or exercising excessively.

There is also a group of eating disorders that do not quite fit into either of the other categories; they used to be called eating disorders not otherwise specified (EDNOS). This group used to lump a bunch of different types of disordered eating into one big category, but it got hard for clinicians to figure out which strategies worked for which kinds of patients (for example, some are called ARFID—avoidant/restrictive food intake disorder). If your doctor is not aware of this diagnosis, seek out a pediatrician and team that are adolescent medicine specialists and/or a group well versed in the treatment of kids with disordered eating. Treatment usually involves a team approach, including doctors, parents, nutritional counselors, and psychological counselors. The therapist ends up serving as a "life coach" or skills builder, helping the person develop better coping strategies so that he or she doesn't use the eating disorder as a default coping mechanism ("I'm stressed, I don't eat; I'm stressed, I overexercise"). This is the opposite from binge eating disorder, which can lead to obesity: "I'm stressed, I eat. I'm stressed, I don't want to exercise." Either way, the person needs new and better skills to handle stress.

Part of overcoming eating disorders is establishing a healthy environment. If you used to enjoy doing an activity with a buddy, try to engage your buddy in the activity, as long as it is a healthful one. Also, avoid "weighty speak"; don't comment on food, body, dieting, or anything weight-related, because the person with the eating disorder is likely to misinterpret whatever you say or find it "triggering," which means it gets her own eating disorder thoughts spiraling out of control.

These are some of the classic signs. Any of them sound familiar? If so, you may need to seek professional help.

- ❏ Preoccupation with appearance, body shape, or weight, with the preoccupation getting in the way of daily life
- ❏ Consistent sadness, frustration, or anger about body image
- ❏ Frequent self-deprecating comments

YOUR STRATEGIES

- ❏ Frequent comparison to others regarding appearance, body shape, or weight
- ❏ Excessive concern about a body part that seems average or okay to others
- ❏ Increasing self-consciousness
- ❏ Secrecy related to eating or exercise habits
- ❏ Dramatic or steady weight loss and/or extreme weight fluctuations (big ups and downs)
- ❏ Severe restriction of food intake
- ❏ Bingeing
- ❏ Refusal to eat certain foods
- ❏ Obsessing over body weight, calories, food, or dieting
- ❏ Unusual eating rituals, such as rearranging food on the plate, excessive chewing, eating food in a certain order, or having to measure all food consumed
- ❏ Making excuses to avoid mealtimes and eating, including claiming food intolerances or allergies when none actually exist
- ❏ Complaining often about feeling fat
- ❏ Excessive exercise, even during bad weather or sickness; feeling the need to get rid of calories consumed
- ❏ Vomiting, diet pills, laxative use, or other forms of purging
- ❏ Frequent weighing
- ❏ Refusal to eat in front of others
- ❏ Consistent denial of hunger
- ❏ Attempts to hide appearance with clothing or posture
- ❏ Moodiness, depression, withdrawn personality

PART 3

THE PLAN

Any smart weight management plan has several components—good eating, good exercise, and good thinking that will help you automate your new behaviors and form them into habits. Above, we've given you the tips and strategies that will serve as the foundation of an approach that will help you lose weight. In this section, we're going to give you more specifics—the ammo you can use to put the principles into play. Below, you'll find:

- ❏ A sample 14-day eating and exercise schedule
- ❏ A sample of recipes that are both easy to make and delicious
- ❏ Three workouts that you can integrate into your week

You can also find much more information, recipes, and strategies in *YOU: On a Diet*, *Cooking the Real Age Way*, and www.realage.com.

THE SAMPLE 14-DAY PLAN

During these two weeks, we'll give you the meal guidelines that can help you change your diet and live it. By the end of the fourteen days, you'll have developed eating patterns and behavioral habits that can help get you on the way to changing your body from the inside out. Here we outline the seven-day plan and strategies for making smart decisions about food and eating. In week two, repeat the first week, making appropriate food substitutions where you wish.

Sunday

Breakfast: Egg-white omelet (no cheese); juice and coffee or tea

Morning snack: Raw veggies

Lunch: Healthful burger with the works

Afternoon snack: Yogurt with fruit

Dinner: Stuffed Whole Wheat Pizza (page 58)

After-dinner exercise: 20-minute walk

Dessert: 1 ounce dark chocolate with a sliced orange

Drinks: Water, coffee, tea, etc., as you wish (see proposed broader list)

Monday

Breakfast: Lifestyle 180 Berry-Banana Smoothie (page 50)

Morning snack: 1 ounce raw nuts

Lunch: Chopped salad of walnuts, veggies, greens, and salmon, turkey, or chicken

Afternoon snack: Yogurt with fruit

Afternoon exercise: 20-minute walk

Dinner: Tofu or Turkey Dogs with Sauerkraut (page 60)

Evening snack: Dry (air-popped) popcorn (not buttered or flavored)

Drinks: Water, coffee, tea, etc., as you wish

Tuesday

Breakfast: Cheerios with skim milk; juice and coffee or tea

Morning snack: Apple

Lunch: Cup of healthful soup; cranberries, walnuts, and crumbled cheese over greens

Afternoon snack: Yogurt with fruit

Dinner: Turkey Tortilla Wraps with Red Baked Potato (page 59)

Dessert: Cinnamon Apple Sauté à la Mode (page 63)

Drinks: Water, coffee, tea, etc., as you wish

Wednesday

Breakfast: Lifestyle 180 Berry-Banana Smoothie (page 50)

Morning snack: 1 ounce raw nuts

Lunch: Chopped salad of walnuts, veggies, greens, and salmon, turkey, or chicken

Afternoon snack: Yogurt and fruit

Dinner: RB's Vegetarian Chili (page 57)

Evening snack: Tomato-Avocado Salsamole and pita toasts (page 62)

Drinks: Water, coffee, tea, etc., as you wish

Thursday

Breakfast: Cheerios with skim milk; juice and coffee or tea

Morning snack: Plum

Lunch: Cup of healthful soup; cranberries, walnuts, and crumbled cheese over greens

Afternoon snack: Raw veggies

Dinner: Leftover chili

Dessert: 1 ounce dark chocolate with a sliced orange

Drinks: Water, coffee, tea, etc., as you wish

Friday

Breakfast: Lifestyle 180 Berry-Banana Smoothie (page 50)

Morning snack: 1 ounce raw nuts

Lunch: Chopped salad of walnuts, veggies, greens, and salmon/turkey/chicken

Afternoon snack: Yogurt with fruit

Dinner: JP's Mac and Cheese (page 56)

Evening snack: Air popped popcorn

Drinks: Water, coffee, tea, etc., as you wish

Saturday

Breakfast: Cheerios with skim milk; juice and coffee or tea

Morning snack: Yogurt with fruit

Lunch: Cup of healthful soup; cranberries, walnuts, and crumbled cheese over greens

Afternoon snack: Raw veggies

Dinner: Experiment! Use our principles and see if you can come up with something fun and healthful. (If not, go back to the Stuffed Whole Wheat Pizza [page 58].)

Dessert: Cinnamon Apple Sauté à la Mode (page 63)

Drinks: Water, coffee, tea, etc., as you wish

SAMPLE RECIPES

We know that you have enough on your plate when it comes to work, school, fun, and all of your other activities. But we also know that it's important to think about what's literally on your plate every day. Too many of us fall into the trap of relying on high-calorie, nonnutritious convenience foods to get us through the day. The fact is that nutrient-rich foods can taste great and be easy to make, and they provide so many more healthful options than overly processed foods. Many of these combos are really simple to make. For example:

Sandwich: Natural peanut butter, blueberries, and/or banana slices on 100 percent whole wheat bread.

Salad: Your favorite vegetables and lettuce topped with black beans and your favorite lean meat (for instance, white meat chicken or turkey); sprinkle lightly with olive oil and lemon juice.

Smoothie: Low-fat or skim milk and/or low-fat or nonfat yogurt, your favorite fruit, and ice in a blender.

Snacks: Grapes on toothpicks frozen for a day or more in the freezer; fresh pea pods, cucumber slices, radishes, carrots, celery, beans, or other veggies with a healthful dip or salsa. You can also make homemade applesauce (peeled apple cut up into chunks or slices, 2 tablespoons water, and some cinnamon; microwave 2 to 3 minutes, check for softness/mushability, microwave another minute and recheck, until you get to the right consistency).

Burger: Just sub in some beans or even chopped veggies for some or most (or even all) of the lean ground meat.

The options are endless, but we also believe there's a lot of value in enjoying the process of preparing healthful foods. So here we offer some fun and healthful recipes. Make them with your family, and enjoy the process of making healthful meals that everyone will enjoy—both because of how they taste and how they make you feel.

Lifestyle 180 Berry-Banana Smoothie
2 servings ❖ 130 calories per serving

1 small banana, broken into chunks

1 cup fat-free plain yogurt

½ cup orange juice

½ cup fresh or frozen raspberries

¼ cup fresh or frozen blueberries

½ cup fresh or frozen blackberries

Combine all the ingredients in a blender. Cover and blend until fairly smooth.

Total fat 0.5 g • Saturated fat 0 g • Healthful fats 0 g • Fiber 4 g •
Carbohydrates 28 g • Sugar 20 g • Protein 6 g • Sodium 65 mg •
Calcium 176 mg • Magnesium 37 mg • Selenium 4 mcg • Potassium 435 mg

Pineapple-Banana Protein Blaster

2 servings ❖ 207 calories per serving

1 large ripe banana, broken into chunks

½ cup low-fat (1 percent) soy milk

1 can (4 ounces) crushed pineapple in juice, undrained

½ cup "pineapple-passion" sorbet, such as Select brand
   (a Safeway brand)

1 tablespoon soy protein powder (8 grams protein)

Combine all the ingredients in a blender. Cover and blend until fairly smooth.

Total fat 2 g • Saturated fat 0.8 g • Healthful fats 1.1 g • Fiber 2.1 g •
Carbohydrates 38 g • Sugar 17 g • Protein 11 g • Sodium 31 mg •
Calcium 39 mg • Magnesium 40 mg • Selenium 1 mcg • Potassium 428 mg

Lifestyle 180 Banana Steel-Cut Oatmeal with Cinnamon

3 servings ❖ 200 calories per serving

2⅓ cups fat-free milk

⅔ cup steel-cut oats

⅛ teaspoon salt

1 large banana, thinly sliced

½ teaspoon ground cinnamon

Place 2 cups of the milk in a medium saucepan. Bring to a gentle simmer over high heat. Stir in the oats and salt. Reduce heat to low; simmer, stirring frequently, until most of the milk is absorbed and the oats are tender, about 25 minutes. Remove from heat; stir in the banana and cinnamon. Pour into two cereal bowls and serve with the remaining ⅓ cup milk.

Total fat 2 g • Saturated fat 0 g • Healthful fats 0 g • Fiber 4 g • Carbohydrates 37 g • Sugar 12 g • Protein 11 g • Sodium 170 mg • Calcium 190 mg • Magnesium 8 mg • Selenium 0 mcg • Potassium 106 mg

Lifestyle 180 Choose Your Fruit Pancakes
Makes 12 to 14 pancakes ❖ 110 calories per serving (2 pancakes)

1⅓ cups whole wheat pastry flour

1 tablespoon baking powder

¾ teaspoon salt

½ teaspoon cinnamon

1 tablespoon ground chia seeds

1⅓ cups water

1 tablespoon vanilla extract

½ cup toasted walnuts

1 apple, grated

1 pear, grated

1 banana, peeled, halved, and thinly sliced

In a large bowl, combine the flour, baking powder, salt, cinnamon, and ground chia seeds and mix well with a wire whisk. In a separate measuring cup, combine the water and vanilla extract. Add the mixture to the dry ingredients and mix well with a wire whisk. Add the walnuts, apple, and pear to the mixture and mix well; then add the banana. Mix well, and if the batter seems a little thick, add 2 tablespoons of water. Make the pancakes in a preheated, nonstick pan that has been wiped with a light film of vegetable oil. Cook over medium heat until brown on both sides and serve.

Total fat 4 g • Saturated fat 0 g • Healthful fats 3.7 g • Fiber 3 g •
Carbohydrates 18 g • Sugar 4 g • Protein 2 g • Sodium 280 mg •
Calcium 49 mg • Magnesium 13 mg • Selenium 0 mcg • Potassium 88 mg

Black Bean Soup
Four 1-cup servings ❖ 105 calories each

1 cup diced onion

1 tablespoon extra-virgin olive oil

2 teaspoons minced fresh garlic

One 15-ounce can black beans, drained and rinsed

½ teaspoon dried oregano

½ teaspoon paprika

¼ teaspoon cumin

2 cups water plus 1 tablespoon natural vegetable base, or 2 cups
    vegetable stock

1 tablespoon canned jalapeño chili peppers, finely chopped

2 tablespoons tomato paste

In a medium pot on medium heat, sauté the onion in the oil until it is transparent. Add the garlic and sauté for two more minutes. Add the remaining ingredients; bring to a simmer and cook for 10 minutes. Turn off the heat, remove the pot from the stove, and stir the soup with a wooden spoon to mix well. Serve or allow the soup to cool and then cover, label, date, and refrigerate.

Total fat 3.3 g • Saturated fat 0.5 g • Healthful fats 2.8 g • Fiber 4.9 g • Carbohydrates 17.5 g • Sugar 2.8 g • Protein 4.3 g • Sodium 275 mg • Calcium 43 mg • Magnesium 8 mg • Potassium 362 mg

Sesame Cucumber Salad

2 servings ❖ 187 calories per serving

1 tablespoon rice wine vinegar

1 teaspoon extra-virgin olive oil

½ teaspoon toasted sesame oil

½ teaspoon soy sauce

Dash of cayenne pepper

2 cucumbers, cut into ¼-inch-thick slices

½ bunch chives, minced

1 teaspoon sesame seeds

Combine the vinegar, olive oil, sesame oil, soy sauce, and cayenne pepper in a medium bowl; mix well. Add the cucumbers, chives, and sesame seeds; mix well and serve.

Total fat 6.8 g • Saturated fat 1 g • Healthful fats 5.3 g • Fiber 3.2 g • Carbohydrates 29 g • Sugar 8.2 g • Protein 6.2 g • Sodium 180 mg • Calcium 90 mg • Magnesium 85 mg • Selenium 18.1 mcg • Potassium 750 mg

Spicy, Crunchy Garlic Broccoli and Cauliflower

Four ½-cup servings ❖ 96 calories each

2 cups small cauliflower florets, fresh or frozen (4 ounces)

2 cups small broccoli florets, fresh or frozen (4 ounces)

2 tablespoons extra-virgin olive oil

1 teaspoon minced fresh garlic

3 tablespoons fresh lemon juice

½ to 1 teaspoon crushed red pepper flakes, as desired

1 teaspoon dried oregano

1 teaspoon minced fresh parsley

½ teaspoon kosher salt

Cook the cauliflower and broccoli florets in a medium saucepan of simmering water for 2 minutes or until still crisp. Drain; rinse with cold water and drain well. Wrap the florets in paper towels and refrigerate. Dry the same saucepan and add the oil and garlic. Sauté the garlic over low heat for 2 minutes or until it is softened. Add the blanched vegetables (the lightly cooked broccoli and cauliflower) and the remaining ingredients to the oil and garlic and toss well. Serve at room temperature, or reheat if you prefer it warm.

Total fat 7.5 g • Saturated fat 1.1 g • Healthful fats 6 g • Fiber 2.5 g •
Carbohydrates 6.3 g • Sugar 1.4 g • Protein 2.2 g • Sodium 266 mg •
Calcium 38 mg • Magnesium 20mg • Potassium 306 mg

JP's Mac and Cheese

Six 1¼-cup servings ❖ 240 calories each

6 ounces elbow macaroni, cavatappi, penne, or rotini 100% whole
wheat pasta (2½ cups dry)

2 medium (14 ounces) sweet potatoes, peeled and diced into ½-inch
cubes, or 14 ounces canned sweet potatoes (no added sugar)

2 cups unsweetened almond milk

6 ounces extra-firm silken tofu

1 teaspoon Dijon mustard

¼ teaspoon ground black pepper

⅛ teaspoon nutmeg

⅛ teaspoon cayenne pepper

4 ounces low-fat shredded mozzarella cheese

Preheat the oven to 350°F. Cook the pasta according to the package directions, omitting the salt. Meanwhile, combine the sweet potatoes and almond milk in a medium saucepan and bring to a boil over high heat. Reduce the heat; simmer, uncovered, until the potatoes are very tender, about 20 minutes. Drain the potatoes, reserving the milk. If the milk measures less than 1½ cups, add additional milk to equal 1½ cups. Purée the sweet potatoes and all of the remaining ingredients except the cheese in a blender until smooth or mash by hand with a wooden spoon, the back of a fork, or a wire whisk. Toss the pasta with the sweet potato sauce and cheese; transfer to an 8- or 9-inch baking dish. Cover with foil; bake for 35 to 40 minutes, or until heated through, and serve.

Total fat 7 g • Saturated fat 3 g • Healthful fats 3.5 g • Fiber 5.2 g •
Carbohydrates 36 g • Sugar 3.7 g • Protein 12 g • Sodium 270 mg •
Calcium 242 mg • Magnesium 53 mg • Potassium 366 mg

RB's Vegetarian Chili

Makes fifteen 1-cup servings ❖ 163 calories each

2 tablespoons canola oil

1 large yellow onion, chopped

4 smashed cloves fresh garlic

1 cup diced carrots

2 large green peppers, roughly chopped

2 jalapeño peppers, seeded and diced

2 medium zucchini, sliced and diced

One 8-ounce bag frozen corn (or 1 cup fresh)

One 8-ounce can tomato paste

One 16-ounce can Muir fire-roasted tomatoes, drained (juice reserved)
and chopped

4 to 5 tablespoons chili powder, or more to taste

2 to 3 tablespoons ground cumin

2 to 3 bay leaves

2 tablespoons dried oregano

Freshly ground pepper (about 15 grinds)

2 chipotle peppers in adobo sauce (these come in a can and
can be found in the ethnic section of the grocery store), chopped

Three 15-ounce cans of red and/or black beans, drained and rinsed

1 cup vegetable stock

In a large, heavy pot, heat the oil over medium-high heat. Add the onion, garlic, and carrots; sauté until the onion is translucent. Add the green peppers and jalapeño peppers, zucchini, and corn; sauté for 5 minutes, stirring occasionally. Add the tomato paste, chopped tomatoes, and tomato juice. Then add the chili powder, cumin, bay leaves, oregano, and pepper. Stir well. Add the chopped chipotle peppers and beans. Stir well. Add the vegetable stock until the liquid covers all of the ingredients in the pot. Bring to a boil; then reduce heat to medium low. Simmer for 30 minutes, stirring occasionally. Remove from heat, adjust the seasonings to taste, and remove the bay leaves. Serve with chopped avocado and fresh lime juice.

Note: This chili is always best the second day. It also goes well with fried or poached eggs for brunch.

Total fat 3.3 g • Saturated fat 0.3 g • Healthful fats 2.9 g • Fiber 7.8 g •
Carbohydrates 27 g • Sugar 5.7 g • Protein 7.5 g • Sodium 431 mg •
Calcium 88 mg • Magnesium 19 mg • Potassium 309 mg

Stuffed Whole Wheat Pizza
4 servings (2 slices per serving) ❖ for the first two weeks, you can have up to half of the pizza, but most people will not need that much to be full at 322 calories per serving

Cooking oil spray

1 pound fresh stir-fry vegetables such as asparagus, broccoli,
    cauliflower, mushrooms, multicolored bell peppers, red and white
    onions, and zucchini, cut up

2 garlic cloves, minced

Salt and freshly ground black pepper (optional)

1 cup pizza sauce or tomato sauce

2 tablespoons olive relish or tapenade

2 tablespoons sundried tomato bits

One 12-inch or 10-ounce prepared thin whole wheat pizza crust
½ cup (2 ounces) finely shredded part-skim mozzarella cheese

Heat the oven to 425°F. Heat a large nonstick skillet over medium-high heat until hot; coat with cooking spray. Add the vegetables and garlic; sauté 2 to 5 minutes, or until the vegetables are crisp-tender. Season to taste with salt and pepper if desired. Combine the pizza sauce, olive relish or tapenade, and sundried tomato bits. Spread over the pizza crust; top with the cooked vegetables and cheese. Bake the pizza directly on the oven rack 10 to 15 minutes, or until the crust is golden brown and the cheese is melted. Cut the pizza into 8 wedges and serve.

Total fat 11.5 g • Saturated fat 3.5 g • Healthful fats 7.9 g • Fiber 5.7 g • Carbohydrates 44.2 g • Sugar 3.5 g • Protein 12.2 g • Sodium 682 mg • Calcium 151 mg • Magnesium 44 mg • Selenium 2.9 mcg • Potassium 481 mg

Turkey Tortilla Wraps with Red Baked Potato
2 servings ❖ 497 calories per serving

Red Potato Ingredients
1 large russet baking potato, washed, pierced with tip of knife
2 tablespoons marinara sauce or other red tomato sauce

Turkey Tortilla Wraps
Two 6-inch whole wheat flour tortillas
4 slices deli roast turkey breast
4 romaine lettuce leaves
4 slices tomato
2 thin slices red or yellow onion
Mustard or hot peppers (optional)

Cook the potato in a microwave on high power 8 to 9 minutes or until fork tender. Slice lengthwise in half and spoon 1 tablespoon sauce over each half. Meanwhile, to prepare the turkey wraps, layer all the turkey wrap ingredients on the tortillas; roll up. Serve together.

Total fat 14.5 g • Saturated fat 4.5 g • Healthful fats 10 g • Fiber 7 g • Carbohydrates 64 g • Sugar 6.5 g • Protein 28.5 g • Sodium 1,654 mg • Calcium 180 mg • Magnesium 71 mg • Selenium 11.3 mcg • Potassium 1,596 mg

Tofu or Turkey Dogs with Sauerkraut
2 servings ❖ 298 calories per serving

4 tofu (meatless) or turkey hot dogs

1 cup sauerkraut

2 tablespoons inexpensive mustard, such as spicy brown or coarse-grained

Whole wheat buns (optional)

Simmer hot dogs in water with sauerkraut until heated through, about 5 minutes. Drain; serve with mustard (with or without buns).

Note: There's a lot of saturated fat here, so we recommend it only as a last-ditch resort.

Total fat 26 g • Saturated fat 9 g • Healthful fats 15.4 g • Fiber 0.7 g • Carbohydrates 3.8 g • Sugar 2.1 g • Protein 11.2 g • Sodium 1,219 mg • Calcium 158 mg • Magnesium 27 mg • Selenium 1.9 mcg • Potassium 160 mg

Lifestyle 180 Chia Sausage or Meatballs
12 servings ❖ 130 calories per serving

¾ cup nonalcoholic red wine

2 tablespoons finely minced garlic

2 tablespoons ground chia seeds

1 tablespoon fennel seed

½ teaspoon dried basil

¼ teaspoon dried oregano

¼ teaspoon dried thyme

¼ teaspoon freshly ground black pepper

2 teaspoons seasoned salt

½ teaspoon crushed red pepper flakes

¼ cup chopped fresh parsley

2 pounds ground turkey breast

In a large bowl, combine the nonalcoholic red wine, garlic, and chia seeds. Set aside and allow the chia seeds to swell for 30 minutes. Add the remaining ingredients except for the turkey and mix well. Add the turkey and mix until well blended. In a large nonstick pan, cook the sausage in either patty form or bulk form until slightly brown and stir to crumble. Drain and serve or cool and refrigerate.

Variation: Makes great Italian meatballs for sandwiches or to go with pasta by adding 2 egg whites and ½ cup bread crumbs to the wine. Scoop or roll into 1-ounce meatballs and place in a shallow baking pan. Bake in a 375°F oven for 20 minutes or to an internal temperature of 165°F. Remove and serve or cool and refrigerate. Yields forty 1-ounce meatballs.

Tips: Use crumbled Italian sausage for pizza toppings, or mix with pasta and your choice of sauce. Milk, broth, V8 juice, or water can be substituted for wine, if desired.

Total fat 2 g • Saturated fat 0 g • Healthful fats 1 g • Fiber 2 g •
Carbohydrates 3 g • Sugar 0 g • Protein 22 g • Sodium 320 mg •
Calcium 38 mg • Magnesium 7.5 mg • Selenium 2 mcg • Potassium 55 mg

Tomato-Avocado Salsamole
2 servings ❖ 90 calories per serving

¼ cup finely chopped red onion

1 teaspoon minced jalapeño, or more to taste

1 tablespoon lime juice

1 tablespoon cider vinegar

1 teaspoon minced garlic

¼ teaspoon salt

1 ripe avocado (preferably Hass), peeled, pitted, and coarsely mashed

1 medium tomato, chopped

¼ cup chopped cilantro

Combine the onion, jalapeño, lime juice, vinegar, garlic, and salt in a bowl. Add the avocado, tomato, and cilantro; mix well. Serve immediately or, to store, reserve avocado pit, add to mixture to prevent browning, cover tightly with plastic wrap, and refrigerate. Serve with lightly toasted whole wheat pita cut into triangles.

Total fat 8 g • Saturated fat 2.1 g • Healthful fats 5.3 g • Fiber 3.1 g •
Carbohydrates 8 g • Sugar 2 g • Protein 2 g • Sodium 25 mg •
Calcium 20 mg • Magnesium 54 mg • Selenium 0 mcg • Potassium 805 mg

Cinnamon Apple Sauté à la Mode

2 servings ❖ 220 calories per serving

2 small apples, such as Jonagold or Ambrosia

1 tablespoon apple butter

1 tablespoon unsweetened apple juice or cider, preferably organic

½ teaspoon ground cinnamon

6 walnut halves, toasted, coarsely chopped

½ cup nonfat or low-fat vanilla frozen yogurt

Cut the apples into quarters; discard the stems, cores, and seeds. Cut the apple quarters into thin slices. Heat a large nonstick skillet over medium-high heat until hot. Add the apples; cook until they begin to brown, about 4 minutes, tossing occasionally. Stir in the apple butter, apple juice, and cinnamon; continue to cook 5 to 8 minutes, or until the apples are tender and the sauce thickens, tossing frequently. Transfer to serving plates and top with nuts. Serve with frozen yogurt.

Total fat 8.4 g • Saturated fat 0.8 g • Healthful fats 7 g • Fiber 6.7 g •
Carbohydrates 38 g • Sugar 27.6 g • Protein 3.6 g • Sodium 23 mg •
Calcium 83 mg • Magnesium 35 mg • Selenium 2 mcg • Potassium 346 mg

Sliced Peaches with Raspberries, Blueberries, and Chocolate Chips

2 servings ❖ 46 calories per serving

2 small ripe peaches, sliced

½ teaspoon ground cinnamon

Pinch of nutmeg

¼ cup (1 ounce) fresh raspberries

¼ cup (1 ounce) fresh blueberries

1½ tablespoons mini semisweet chocolate chips

Combine the peaches with the cinnamon and nutmeg; transfer to two serving plates. Top the peaches with the raspberries, blueberries, and chocolate chips.

Total fat 0.4 g • Saturated fat 0.1 g • Healthful fats 0.28 g • Fiber 2.6 g • Carbohydrates 11.5 g • Sugar 8.9 g • Protein 1 g • Sodium 0.5 mg • Calcium 22 mg • Magnesium 11.5 mg • Selenium 0.1 mcg • Potassium 202 mg

BODY WEIGHT STRENGTH WORKOUT: NO EQUIPMENT REQUIRED

Perform all the exercises in a row once through. This workout helps strengthen and stretch your body. See www.doctoroz .com for videos of workouts.

1. Crisscross
Builds heart strength, helps improve coordination.

With your feet shoulder width apart and your hands on your waist, jump your feet into a crisscross position. Go back and forth, switching your feet from back to front. Do for 30 seconds. For a more advanced exercise, hold your arms out at shoulder height, palms up, and imagine you are holding glasses of water on your palms. As you crisscross, try not to move your hands, so that you don't spill the water.

2. Ground to Sky
Improves balance and strengthens every muscle.

Balancing on one foot, reach down and touch the ground with both hands. Then reach up toward the sky while simultaneously swinging one foot up in front of you, ideally bringing your knee into line with your hip. Do 10 times on each leg.

3. Hamstring Hang
Stretches the hamstrings and back.

With your feet wider than shoulder width apart and your toes pointed forward, slowly drop your hands toward the ground between your feet. Hold for 10 seconds. Walk your hands to your left foot and hold for 10 seconds, then to your right foot and hold for 10 seconds. Move back to the center for 10 seconds. Really relax your neck and think about hanging down instead of reaching down. Take deep breaths the entire time.

4. Armcopter
Stretches the shoulders and gets the blood flowing in the arms.

With your feet together, circle your arms 5 times. Try to clap your hands in front of your face. Your goal is to make the circles as big as feels comfortable. Relax your shoulders and resist bobbing your neck; keep your head upright. Do 2 times.

5. Air Angels
Strengthens the entire back.

Lie facedown on the floor. Close your eyes and reach your arms above your head, your palms facing down. With your feet together, lift your legs off the ground and keep them there. Keeping your arms straight, reach your hands back toward your hips. Go back and forth 25 times, making an angel.

For a more advanced exercise, move your legs as well. The higher you lift your knees and armpits, the harder it will be.

6. Triceps Push-ups
Works the triceps and chest.

While on your stomach, bring your hands underneath your shoulders, your palms down and fingers spread. Kick your heels up so your legs are at right angles, and cross your ankles. Keeping a straight line between the top of your head and your knees, do 20 push-ups. Keep your elbows flush against your sides so that they rub against your shirt. Keep your abs tight. For a more advanced exercise, balance on your toes rather than on your knees.

7. Donkey Kicks
Strengthens the quadriceps and shoulders.

On all fours with your shoulders over your hands and your hips over your knees, lift your knees one inch off the ground. Now bounce and lift your feet one inch off the ground. Do 25 times. Try to float your feet off the ground, and make as little noise as possible. Do 25 times. For a more advanced exercise, try to kick your feet up behind you like a donkey while maintaining a soft landing.

8. Quad Bend
Stretches the quads and knees.

Kneel and position your feet and knees a little wider apart than your hips. Maintain a straight line with the outsides of your lower legs and point your toes directly behind you with the soles of your feet facing up. Drop your tailbone between your heels; lower yourself only as far as feels comfortable for your knees, or else drop all the way down and lie down on your back. Hold for 30 seconds. Scan your body and take deep breaths, releasing any tension.

9. Zigzag
Strengthens the entire core.

Lie on your back with your legs bent and your feet flat on the ground. Interweave your fingers behind your head. Open your elbows to the side so you cannot see them. Lift your head off the ground and hold it there; maintain a relaxed neck. Lift your feet an inch off the ground and zigzag them out until they are almost straight. Go out only as far as you can, keeping your lower back flat on the ground. Then zigzag them back toward your tailbone. Do 20 zigzags.

10. Back Bend
Stretches the abs and chest.

Kneel and place your palms on your back with your fingers pointing down. Looking up toward the ceiling, bring your elbows toward each other. To increase the stretch, gently press your hips forward. Take 5 deep chest breaths.

11. Break Dancing
Strengthens the entire body; great for agility.

Get into the "up" push-up position. Walk your feet around clockwise toward the outside of your left hand. When you get to your left hand, lift it off the ground, walk under it, and put it back on the exact same spot. Keep walking your feet around in front of you until you get to your right hand. When you do, lift it off the ground, walk under it, and put it back on the exact same spot. Do 5 clockwise circles, then 5 counterclockwise. Focus on always having your middle finger pointed up and your elbows barely bent.

Variation: For a more advanced exercise, do it faster.

12. One-Foot Hop
Improves balance; strengthens the legs; improves cardio.

With your hands on your waist and balancing on one foot with your standing leg slightly bent, hop around in circles 5 times; switch directions and do 5 more times. Do 2 times. For a more advanced exercise, do a shoulder press on every hop. Resist looking down; look straight ahead.

13. Invisible Chair
Stretches the hips and lower back; improves balance.

Standing in place, lift your right ankle up on top of your left quad. With your hands on your waist, slowly lower your tailbone until you get a stretch in your hip. Hold for 20 seconds; switch sides and repeat. Take long, deep breaths throughout the stretch.

Variation: For a more advanced exercise, straighten your arms above your head, palms facing inward, and bring your thumbs back as you squat lower.

BAND WORKOUT

Some people use dumbbells to work out. Others use barbells. Some (including us) use their own body weight. Another great way to work and tone your muscles is with resistance bands. These stretchy bands offer various amounts of resistance, so that you can push, pull, and move to test all the muscles of your body. We recommend that you do the following workout, designed by trainer Joel Harper, two or three times a week.

Follow these guidelines for the workout:

1. Use a band with handles, and always grip the handles firmly.
2. Choose a band that you can use comfortably throughout the entire workout. As soon as that becomes easy, use a thicker band, or, for certain exercises, wrap the band around your hands.
3. Keep the band away from your face.
4. If you find the band uncomfortable on your skin, wear a long-sleeved shirt.
5. Breathe normally and stand upright.
6. When tightening the band, wrap it around your hand, not the handle.

Warm-up: Figure Eight

Warms up the shoulders and arms.

Stand with your feet shoulder width apart and circle your

arms and hands together in figure eights down, around, up, and across to the other side. Do 8 times.

1. Standing Chest Press
Warms up and strengthens your chest and arms.

Grab both handles and place the band behind your back, just underneath your shoulder blades. Wrap the band around your hands to shorten it. With your hands out to your sides at shoulder height, act as if you're hugging a tree and bring your hands together in front of you on the exhale. Inhale and bring your hands back to your sides. Do 25 times.

Advanced: Do 50 times and work your calves by rising up on the balls of your feet as you bring your arms together.

2. Standing Chest Pull
Strengthens your chest and arms.

Stand on the band with your feet shoulder width apart. Hold the band down by your sides, then slowly lift your right hand (palm side up) out in front of the right side of your chest, then lower it. Move your left hand up and back down; do 25 times for each arm. If this is easy for you, do both at the same time.

Advanced: After you're done, hold both hands at the highest point for 30 seconds with palms facing up.

3. Chest Opener
Stretches your chest and arms.

Leave the band loosely in your hands and interweave your fingers behind your head without touching your head. While standing upright, act as if there are strings on your elbows and hands, pulling them directly behind you, as you take five breaths deep into your chest.

4. *Lateral Raise*
Strengthens your shoulders.

Holding the handles with your hands at your sides and your palms down, lift your arms straight out to your sides 25 times, always leading with your elbows, not your wrists.

Advanced: After you're done, hold the handles up for 30 seconds.

5. *Neck Stretch*
Opens the neck.

With your hands hanging down to your sides and your shoulders level, gently drop your right ear down toward your right shoulder. Let go of all the tension in your body. Hold for three deep breaths; switch sides and repeat.

6. *Lateral Circle*
Strengthens your shoulders and rotator cuffs.

Standing on the band and holding the handles, reach your arms out to your sides and bring your hands up as high as you can but not more than shoulder height. Rotate clockwise the size of a cantaloupe 25 times; then switch directions and repeat.

7. *Chicken Wing*
Stretches your shoulders.

Without the band, place the back side of your right hand just above your right hip. Standing up straight, take your left hand and clasp your right elbow behind you (if you can't, slide your right hand behind your lower back until you can reach your elbow). Gently pull your elbow toward your belly button and take 5 deep breaths into your upper chest, opening the tightest area. Keep your chest lifted and your shoulders even. Switch sides and repeat.

8. *Lateral Pull-Down*
Strengthens your upper back and arms.

With your feet together, wrap the band around each hand 3 times. Lift your hands above your head with your palms facing forward. With straight arms, pulse your hands away from each other 25 times, keeping the band taut the entire time.

Advanced: Do 25 times balancing on your left foot with your right knee in line with your right hip; switch sides and repeat.

9. *Lateral Hold*
Strengthens your upper back and arms; builds stamina.

Hold the band above your head with your hands apart for 25 seconds with the band as tight as possible. Don't tighten your face or scrunch your shoulders.

Advanced: Do the exercise while balancing on your toes.

10. *Shoulder Height*
Strengthens your upper back and arms.

With your hands holding the handles at shoulder height and your arms straight out in front of you, pulse your hands away from each other 25 times.

Advanced: Do the above, simultaneously bringing one knee to hip height. While keeping your knee stationary, swing your lower leg from side to side. Do 25 times; switch sides and repeat.

11. *Palms Out*
Opens your upper back and shoulders.

Without the band, interweave your fingers and turn your palms away from your body (so you're looking at your knuckles). Reach your palms as far away from you as possible as you hunch your back and curl your tailbone under. Take 5 deep breaths, expanding your rib cage.

12. *Side Triceps Extension*
Strengthens your triceps.

Holding the handles in both hands, wrap the band around your left hand only and reach both hands out to your sides to shoulder height. Take your right hand with your palm facing forward and, leaving your elbow stationary, bring your hand toward your chest 25 times; switch sides and repeat.

Advanced: Balance on one foot and wrap the band around one more time.

13. *Arm Circle*

Warms up your biceps.

Stand with both feet on the band and hold the handles. Reach your hands out to your sides, palm side up, and reach your arms out as high as you can. Do 25 cantaloupe-size circles; then switch direction and repeat.

14. *Side Curl*

Strengthens your biceps.

Holding the band handles with your hands down at your sides, turn your thumbs as far back as feels comfortable. Curl your arms up 25 times. Resist bringing your arms to the front.

Advanced: Do 50 in double time.

15. *Going to Jail*

Opens your shoulders and arms.

Without the band, interweave your fingers behind your tailbone. With your chest lifted, arms straight, and shoulders down, lift your fingers toward the ceiling. Resist rolling your shoulders forward.

Advanced: Bend forward, drop your forehead down toward your shins, and press your knuckles toward the ground.

16. *Penguin*

Strengthens your butt and entire leg.

Stand on the band and hold the handles. Bring your hands

up to elbow height. Keep your hands open and facing up (don't squeeze the handles). Step your right foot to your right, plant it, then bring your left foot over to it. Then step your left foot to the left and bring your right foot over to it. Go back and forth 25 times.

Advanced: Lift your leading foot off the ground and tilt your body from side to side.

17. *Cross Leg Drop*
Stretches your back and hamstrings.

Without the band, cross your left foot over your right. Ideally, you want your big toes in line, but go to where you feel comfortable balancing. Slowly walk your hands down your legs as far as feels comfortable; really relax your neck, as if your head were a bowling ball elongating your spine, and take 3 deep breaths into your back; switch sides and repeat.

18. *Squat*
Strengthens and tones your entire leg.

Holding the handles in front of you with the band under both feet and your feet shoulder width apart, drop down as far as feels comfortable, as if you were sitting in a chair. As you squat, reach your arms straight out in front of you at shoulder height. Come all the way back up to slightly bent knees. Do 25 times.

Advanced: In the squat position, pulse 25 times.

19. Butt Blaster
Tones the butt.

Get on all fours and wrap the band underneath your right heel with the handles underneath both hands. Kick your right heel back 25 times; switch sides and repeat. Really focus on squeezing your butt and lifting your leg every time. Look slightly above your hands during the movement.

Advanced: Do 50 times each leg and pulse at the highest movement 25 times.

20. Thread the Needle
Stretches your hips and lower back.

Without the band, lie on your back. With your knees bent, place your right leg on your left thigh just above the knee. Reach your hands up and through your legs and clasp your left leg. Pull your knees slightly toward your chin and press your tailbone back down to the mat. Resist overarching your neck; keep it straight and relax down on the mat. Take 3 deep breaths; switch sides and repeat.

21. Cross-Legged Lift
Strengthens your lower abs.

Lying on your back without the band, cross your right leg on top of your left with your right ankle against your left thigh and your hands behind your head, your fingers interwoven. Lift your legs slightly, using your lower abs, and set your left foot back down. Do 25 times; switch sides and repeat.

Advanced: Really lift your tailbone off the ground and crunch your upper and lower body with your leg going higher in the air. Do 25 times on each side.

22. *Cross-Legged Twist*
Strengthens your obliques and abs.

Without the band, on your back with your right leg crossed over as in Thread the Needle, place your left hand behind your head and your right hand on your stomach as a sensor to keep it from lifting. Using your core, twist 25 times; switch sides and repeat. Focus on keeping your face relaxed, your chin away from your chest, and your elbows out of your line of vision.

Advanced: Do the exercise with your left leg straight up toward the ceiling 25 times; switch sides and repeat.

23. *Spinal Twist*
Opens your hips, back, and spine.

Without the band, lie on your back with your hands behind your head, your fingers interwoven. With your knees bent and your feet flat on the ground while exhaling, slowly drop your knees to the right and look straight up at the ceiling. To increase the stretch, lift your knees a little higher. Keep your upper back and shoulders on the mat throughout entire pose. Hold for 30 seconds; switch sides and repeat.

THE YOGA WORKOUT

You don't have to be a human rubber band to appreciate the beauty of yoga. This ancient practice not only stretches your muscles but also allows your mind to focus and trains your brain for meditation. The beauty of this workout is that people of any skill level can participate; you need to move only as far into each pose as you can. In fact, the only imperative you have to remember is our golden rule for yoga, which is to take deep belly breaths, using your diaphragm to pull the lungs down during inspiration. (If the poses we outline below are too difficult for you to take continuous deep breaths, back off to avoid compromising this golden rule.) That's important because most of us never take a single deep breath all day long. To exhale, suck your belly button toward your spine to push the diaphragm up and empty all the air from your lungs. Inhaling deeply brings a chemical called nitric oxide from the back of your nose and your sinuses into your lungs. This short-lived gas dilates the air passages in your lungs and the blood vessels surrounding those air passages so you can get more oxygen into your body. Nitric oxide also doubles as a neurotransmitter to help your brain function. Other benefits of yoga:

❑ Yoga and the deep breathing associated with it help
   create a negative pressure in your lungs, acting as a
   vacuum cleaner to draw lymphatic drainage back into
   your veins. What are lymphatics? When your tissues are
   fed by blood, some of the waste material seeps out into
   spaces between cells and becomes lymph. Your lymph

nodes serve as a portal to pass waste material back into your blood vessels for cleansing; these same nodes get inflamed when we are sick, which is why you can feel them getting enlarged. Yoga stimulates the flow in your lymphatic system by exercising your muscles and through the vacuum action of deep breathing.

❑ Yoga trains you to loosen the muscles and joints that are ignored in your day-to-day life. The routines get the blood flowing as you warm up and free your body to experience the stresses you will inevitably face each day. The practice also helps you handle the weight of your body more effectively, which builds bone and muscle strength so you are more resilient. And it improves your balance so you don't fall.

❑ Yoga also helps you to focus your mind on remote parts of your body, such as tight joints and muscles, as you gently but firmly deepen into your poses. Attaining the "empty" mind called for in meditation is difficult, especially for novices, because the mind wanders. But if you can concentrate on the tension in your hip, for example, as you focus your mind on your pose, you're well on your way. The goal in yoga is not really to empty the mind but rather to free the mind to let any and all ideas pass through it rapidly without any attachment.

This workout is a process of self-realization and is designed to help you feel empowered and build your self-discipline. Follow these guidelines to improve your yoga experience.

- ❏ Never force a pose so you feel a painful strain. Go only to where it feels comfortable.
- ❏ If your knees feel discomfort, use a rolled-up towel, pillow, or blanket as a cushion behind the knee joint (in the popliteal area, if you know where that is).
- ❏ Resist locking your elbows.
- ❏ If a pose is difficult to balance, stand against the wall. Your balance may be different from one day to the next. Imbalance during poses may mean an imbalance in other parts of your life.

1. Standing Twist
Warms up your spine; loosens your body.

With your feet shoulder width apart (mountain pose) and your knees slightly bent with relaxed arms, twist your upper body loosely from side to side. Look where you are going. Breathe normally for 30 seconds.

2. Standing Leaning Stretch
Opens your lower back and obliques.

Interweave the fingers of your hands and turn your hands palm side up above your head. Inhale and exhale deeply as you stretch to the right; inhale, come back to the center, and exhale as you stretch to the left. Do 5 times.

3. X
Warms up your upper body.

With your feet in the mountain pose, bring your arms up straight toward the ceiling in a V shape with the palms facing each other. Inhale, and on the exhale, cross your hands in front of your face, bringing your hands to shoulder height with the palms facing you. Inhale; then exhale and cross your arms again, switching the arm closest to you. The exhale should be sharp and come from your navel. Do continuously for 90 seconds, alternating your arms.

4. Ladybug

Opens your upper back, neck, and lungs.

Inhale deeply and place your fingertips on your shoulders with your elbows out to the sides in line with your shoulders. Keeping your fingers on your shoulders, on the exhalation, bring your elbows out in front; keep exhaling and drop your head, bend forward at the neck, and look down to your toes. On the inhale, come back to where your elbows are out to the side. Repeat 5 times.

5. Tightrope

Improves balance; strengthens your ankles.

With your feet in the mountain pose, bring your hands, palm side up, out to your sides at shoulder height. Lift your heels off the ground and balance on your toes. Hold for 30 seconds, taking deep breaths from your navel up into your chest.

Advanced: Do it with your eyes closed.

6. Tree

Improves balance.

With your hands in the prayer position (thumbs against

your chest) and your feet together, slide your right foot up your leg, placing the sole of the foot flush against the leg. Lift your foot as high as you feel comfortable, bringing your knee into line with your hip, and hold for 30 seconds; switch sides and repeat.

Advanced: Interweave your fingers and stretch your hands, palm side up, above your head.

7. *Stork*
Improves balance and focus; strengthens your arms, shoulders, and legs.

While in the mountain pose, bring your right knee up into line with your right hip or as high as 90 degrees. With your right toes pointing toward the floor, inhale and raise your arms straight in front of you, palms facing up, to shoulder height. Resist leaning forward; keep your standing leg pressing into the ground, stand erect, and gaze straight ahead at a fixed point. Hold the pose for 30 seconds and return to the mountain pose; switch sides and repeat.

8. *Horse*
Strengthens your quadriceps and knees.

With your feet wide and your toes turned out 45 degrees, bend your knees so that they're directly above your heels; bring your hands center and into the prayer position. Squat down as low as feels comfortable, but with your tailbone no lower than your knees. Feel the length of your spine by elongating the distance from your tailbone to the top of your head. Hold the pose for 30 seconds.

9. *Goddess*

Strengthens your quadriceps and knees; opens your chest; increases arm strength.

While in the Horse pose, extend your arms out to the side with your elbows slightly below your shoulders. With your palms facing up, bend your elbows to a 90-degree angle. With your palms facing your ears, hold for 30 seconds. Relax into the pose. Don't raise your shoulders; keep them lowered and relaxed.

10. *Triangle*

Opens your spine; helps balance your body.

Stand with your right foot pointing directly to the right and your left foot pointing forward at a slight angle. Inhale deeply. As you exhale, move your right hand down your leg toward your right ankle, stopping wherever you feel comfortable, and simultaneously lift your left hand above your head with the palm facing forward. Look up at your left hand, keeping your shoulder parallel to your hip the entire time. Resist twisting your shoulders. Take 5 deep breaths; switch sides and repeat. Do 2 times.

11. *Cat Back/Cow*

Improves the flexibility of your spine and circulation in your torso.

Get down on all fours with your weight evenly distributed; keep your knees under your hips and your wrists under your shoulders. Your arms are straight but not locked, and your fingers are spread and facing forward. Start with a straight line from the top of your head to your tailbone. Exhale as you lift your upper back, tuck your tailbone underneath, and look toward your belly button, tucking your chin in. Inhale as you reverse into the cow position and lift your tailbone up; your belly button goes toward the ground. Look straight ahead as the top of your head faces the ceiling. Use your entire spine throughout the movement. Do 5 times.

12. Extended Cat Stretch
Warms up and awakens your entire body; great for your spine.

While in the Cat Back pose, lift your left knee off the ground and bring it toward your forehead while simultaneously tucking your forehead under. Then inhale and smoothly extend your right leg behind you with pointed toes. Lift your head and look forward. During the entire movement, keep your hips in line and your pelvis steady as you elongate your entire body. Do 5 times; switch sides and repeat.

13. Thread the Needle
Opens your upper back and shoulders.

Start on all fours; take your right hand palm side down and slide it under your left armpit. Keep extending it as you exhale and slowly lower your right ear and shoulder to the mat. Simultaneously drop your left elbow onto the mat or as low as feels comfortable. Hold for 30 seconds; switch sides and repeat.

14. Lion
Awakens and simultaneously relaxes your facial muscles.

While on your knees, sit erect and take a deep inhale. On the exhale, stretch all your facial muscles apart, open your mouth as wide as you can, try to touch your tongue to your chin, and open your hands as wide as you can with palms facing out. Look at the tip of your nose and make a loud "Ha!" sound. Do 4 times.

15. *Wrist Extensions*
Opens your wrists; helps with carpal tunnel problems.

Bring your hands out in front of you chest high, palm side down, and interweave your fingers. Relax your shoulders and gently pull your elbows apart, creating space in your joints. Keeping this space, raise your left wrist and lower your right, keeping both forearms parallel to the ground. Now your right wrist is bending up and your left wrist is bending down. Keeping your fingers interlaced, gently go back and forth several times, opening up your wrists and switching your leading hand.

16. *Camel*
Opens your chest and the front of your body; strengthens your spine.

While on your knees (use a folded towel under them if needed), place your knees and feet 6 inches apart. Place your hands on the back of your hips, fingers pointed down. Drop your head back completely and support yourself with your hands. Take a deep breath and exhale as you press your thighs, hips, and stomach forward, using your spinal strength. While taking deep breaths, hold the bend for 20 seconds and come out slowly.

17. Yoga Lunges

Stretches your thighs and groin; lengthens your spine.

On all fours with your knees below your hips and your hands below your shoulders, step your left foot forward, placing it next to your left hand. Your left shin stays perpendicular to the ground; on the inhale, bring both your hands up onto your left thigh. Keep the front of your knee behind your big toe. Don't raise your shoulders toward your ears; keep them broad. If this is too hard, leave one hand down until it feels easy and then come up. On the exhale, gently twist your right hip toward your left heel, so that you feel a stretch along your back thigh. Inhale and exhale 4 times; switch sides and repeat.

18. Down Dog

Strengthens and stretches your legs and shoulders; energizes your whole body.

Start on all fours with your hands shoulder width apart and your feet hip width apart. Tuck your toes under. While inhaling, lift your knees off the ground and straighten your legs. Lift your hips back and up and spread your fingers out, pressing your palms flat to the floor. Keep your neck relaxed; your head should be in a neutral position. Lift your quadriceps muscles; keep them activated. Draw your heels toward the floor. Hold for 30 seconds and release back down to the mat while exhaling.

19. Cobra

Develops strength and flexibility in your back.

Lie on your stomach with your hands palm side down under your shoulders, keeping your fingertips directly underneath the tops of your shoulders. Your legs are together and tight like a rock. Point your toes and put your elbows flush against your sides. While looking up at the ceiling, use your spine strength and lift your torso off the floor just to the navel. Resist pressing with your hands, and arch your back as much as feels comfortable. Keep your shoulders relaxed and down away from your ears. Hold for 20 seconds.

20. Diagonal Reach
Strengthens your back with emphasis on your lower back and butt; improves coordination.

Lying on your stomach, place your right hand, palm down, underneath your relaxed forehead. Bring your left straight arm beside your left ear, then lift it off the ground while simultaneously lifting your right leg. Focus on stretching the fingers of your left hand as far as you can away from your right foot, and feel your whole body lengthening. It is more important to elongate than to lift higher. Hold for 20 seconds; switch sides and repeat. Do 2 times on each side.

21. Half Frog Pose
Stretches your quadriceps; great for your knees.

Lie facedown and rest your forehead on the back of your left hand. Lift your right foot toward your right hip and grab your foot with your right hand. Pull the foot gently toward your outer hip. Breathe evenly and hold for 30 seconds; release, switch sides and repeat.

22. Down Dog One Leg

Strengthens and stretches the legs; stretches your calves; energizes your whole body.

In the Down Dog pose, take your right foot off the ground and wrap it around your left ankle. This added weight will open up your calf. Hold for 15 seconds; switch sides and repeat.

23. Roll and Massage Back

Massages your back; improves balance.

Lying on your back, bend your knees and clasp your hands onto your hamstrings. Curl your tailbone up and round your back. Rock back and forth as much as feels comfortable, taking notice of any skips in your roll. Try to round your body as much as possible, so it rocks smoothly back and forth. Use your lower legs to swing your body. Do for 30 seconds.

24. Little Boat Pose

Stretches your hips, lower back, and spine.

Lying on your back, hug your knees in toward your chest with your hands. Release your left leg down (either straight or bent, whichever feels more comfortable) and interweave your fingers on the outside of your right leg, just underneath the knee. Slightly pull the right knee in toward your right shoulder as you relax your neck and keep your shoulders down. Resist overextending your neck; elongate it and look straight up. Hold for 30 seconds; switch sides and repeat.

25. Little Boat Twist

Stretches your hips, lower back, and spine.

On your back, reach your arms straight out to shoulder height, flush against the ground, palm side down. With your knees bent and feet flat on the ground, exhale as you slowly drop your knees to the right and look straight up at the ceiling. To increase the stretch, lift your knees a little higher. Keep your upper back and shoulders on the mat throughout the entire pose. Hold for 30 seconds; switch sides and repeat.

26. Half Boat
Tones your stomach and back.

Sit on the floor. Keeping your knees bent and together out in front of you and your hands holding your thighs lean back to about a 45-degree angle. Slowly bring your feet off the ground with your calves parallel to the ground and balance. When you have your balance, release your hands to knee height.

Advanced: Straighten your legs into a V shape. Hold for 30 seconds.

27. Butterfly
Opens your hips and groin.

Sit on the floor with your knees bent and the soles of your feet together. Interweave your fingers on the outsides of your feet and draw your heels comfortably in toward your tailbone. If this is too hard, place your hands on your legs. With your back straight, slowly tilt your upper body forward. With time and as your hips loosen, you will ultimately be able to drop your chin down on the other side of your toes. Hold for 30 seconds.

28. *Half Butterfly*
Stretches your back, hamstrings, and calves.

Sitting erect on the floor with your legs out in front of you, bend your left leg back into the Half Butterfly pose. Flex your right foot up (resist contorting your foot); keep it straight as if there were a board below it. Walk your hands down your right leg, slowly lowering your forehead toward your right knee. Stop wherever it feels comfortable. Hold for 10 seconds, taking deep breaths into your rib cage; switch sides and repeat.

Advanced: Pull your toes back with your opposite hand.

29. *Corpse*
Relaxes your entire body.

While on your back, let your arms relax down to your sides with your palms facing up, extend your legs out straight, and let your feet flop outward. With your eyes closed, travel mentally throughout your entire body, relaxing from your toes to the crown of your head. Cover your eyes with a cloth if you like. When you are ready to come up, roll onto your side, hold for 15 seconds, then slowly come up onto all fours before standing up.

The 24 Best Health Tips for Teens

Being a proper weight is only part of the equation of being healthy (though it's a very big part, for sure). An overall approach—and managing all areas of wellness—is the best bet for raising a teen who will turn into a healthy and happy adults. Below are our 24 best health tips for teens (you can find elaboration on any of these topics in: *YOU: The Owner's Manual for Teens*).

1. Realize that you control what goes into your body. Realize that it's never too late to start adopting healthy habits. You get a do-over.
2. Walk ten thousand steps (about five miles) a day.
3. Have one buddy who shares your ideals about living a healthy lifestyle and who you're comfortable talking with about healthy habits.
4. Avoid known toxins such as tobacco, bisphenol A (BPA) in plastics, and toxins found in dry cleaning and some cosmetic products. That means stay away from formaldehyde (found in some Brazilian Blowout products, "smoking water," and embalming fluid).
5. Avoid the five food felons: saturated fats, trans fats,

added sugar, added syrup, non–100 percent whole grains.

6. Eat cruciferous vegetables such as broccoli, cabbage, cauliflower, watercress, and arugula three times a week.

7. Take half a multivitamin twice every day, and get your recommended daily amount of calcium through food or supplements as well as vitamin D3 and DHA omega-3 fats (200 mg a day).

8. Floss and brush your teeth for at least two minutes twice a day.

9. Keep your waist size equal to less than half your height (in inches).

10. Sleep eight and a half to nine hours a night (in greater than ninety-minute blocks).

11. Do some kind of exercise nearly every day, including some form of resistance exercise and cardiovascular exercise.

12. Do one small (or big) form of stress management every day.

13. Have your vaccinations against major diseases up to date.

14. Commit to not texting and driving.

15. Keep your phone and other devices out of your hands (and away from your eyes) while driving (or walking, if you're in urban areas).

16. Have a passion. And do it as often as you can! Safely.

17. Protect your ears from noise louder than a lawn mower (including keeping your personal device on less than 70 percent of max when using earphones).

18. Find a mentor.
19. Practice smart Internet and texting safety, knowing that what you write or post can be saved forever (or posted publicly forever), and be smart about whom you communicate with.
20. Make sex a choice, not something that "just happens." Your body is yours to do what you want with it. If you want it to be a toy for someone else, that is your choice. If you want sex to be a meaningful thing, that is also your choice. And if you are considering becoming sexually active (whether you're a guy or a girl), remember to always carry a condom. And use a second method of contraception if you're having heterosexual sex.
21. Eliminate processed foods from your diet and substitute 100 percent whole wheat flour for white flour where you can.
22. Eat five servings of fruits and veggies per day. Eat fruit but skip the juice unless you are trying to gain weight.
23. Don't squeeze zits.
24. Wear a helmet every time (no excuses) when cycling, Roller Blading, skiing, snowboarding, skateboarding, or rock climbing, and wear a seat belt whenever you're in a car.

INDEX

Air Angels (strength exercise), 65–66

amino acids, 8. *See also specific amino acid*

anorexia nervosa (AN), 41

appetite
  biology and, 9–11, 13, 17
  strategies for weight loss and, 30, 33

Arm Circle (band exercise), 74

Armcopter (strength exercise), 65

athletes, 27

automation
  components of weight management plans and, 45
  strategies for weight loss and, 27–29

Back Bend (strength exercise), 67

band workout, 69–77
  Arm Circle, 74
  Butt Blaster, 76
  Chest Opener, 70–71
  Chicken Wing, 72
  Cross Leg Drop, 75
  Cross-Legged Lift, 76–77
  Cross-Legged Twist, 77
  Figure Eight Warm-up, 69–70
  Going to Jail, 74
  guidelines for, 69
  Lateral Circle, 71
  Lateral Hold, 72
  Lateral Pull-Down, 72
  Lateral Raise, 71
  Neck Stretch, 71
  Palms Out, 73
  Penguin, 74–75
  Shoulder Height, 73

  Side Curl, 74
  Side Triceps Extension, 73
  Spinal Twist, 77
  Squat, 75
  Standing Chest Press, 70
  Standing Chest Pull, 70
  Thread the Needle, 76

behavior: impact of environment on, 23–24

bingeing, 41
  biology and, 12–13
  biology of emotions and, 15
  eating disorders and, 41, 42, 43
  exercise, 38, 43
  strategies for weight loss and, 38

biology
  of emotions, 15–21
  fat and, 5–24
  of the heart, 14–15
  of hunger, 7–11
  and impact of environmental change on behavior, 23
  influence of environment on, 23–24
  of movement, 11–13
  of muscles, 13–14
  reasons for weight gain and, 22
  and weight loss, 21–24
  weight management and, 2–3

bisphenol A (BPA), 91

Black Bean Soup (recipe), 53–54

blood pressure, 7, 37

blood sugar, 6

body mass index (BMI), 22

brain
  biology of emotions and, 16–18
  biology of movement and, 13

brain (*continued*)
    eating disorders and, 40, 41
    strategies for weight loss and,
        26–27, 30–31
    undereating and, 26–27
    See also hypothalamus; *specific
        chemical*
Break Dancing (strength exercise),
    67–68
breakfast
    biology of movement and, 12
    sample meal plans for, 46–48
    skipping, 12
    strategies for weight loss and, 29
buddies: health tips about, 91
bulimia nervosa (BN), 41
burgers: recipes for, 50
Butt Blaster (band exercise), 76
Butterfly (yoga exercise), 89

caffeine, 38
calcium, 92
calories
    ballparking number of, 27
    counting of, 27
    eating disorders and, 41
    exercise and, 36, 37
    obsessing about, 27, 28
    required number of, 27
    strategies for weight loss and, 27,
        28, 30, 36, 37
Camel (yoga exercise), 85
carbohydrates
    automating eating and, 28
    biology of emotions and, 18
    biology of hunger and, 7, 8
    function of, 8
    reasons for weight gain and, 22
    sources of, 7, 25, 26
    strategies for weight loss and, 25,
        26, 28, 33–34
    cardiovascular exercise, 37, 92
Cat Back/Cow (yoga exercise), 83–84
cell phones: driving and, 92
cerebral cortex, 30
Chest Opener (band exercise), 70–71

Chicken Wing (band exercise), 72
cholesterol, 5–6, 7
Cinnamon Apple Sauté à la Mode
    recipe for, 63
    sample 14-day meal plan and,
        47, 48
Cobra (yoga exercise), 86–87
control
    biology of emotions and, 20–21
    eating disorders and, 41
    health tips about, 91
Corpse (yoga exercise), 90
cortisol, 16–18
cravings
    biology of emotions and, 15, 17,
        20
    biology of hunger and, 11
    and impact of environmental
        change on behavior, 23
    reasons for weight gain and, 22
Crisscross (strength exercise), 64
Cross Leg Drop (band exercise), 75
Cross-Legged Lift (band exercise),
    76–77
Cross-Legged Twist (band exercise),
    77
cycling, 93

depression: biology of emotions and,
    16
deprivation diets, 7, 12, 14, 26–27.
    See also undereating
desserts: sample 14-day plan for,
    46–48
diabetes, 7
Diagonal Reach (yoga exercise), 87
dining out, 24
dinner: sample 14-day plan for,
    46–48
Donkey Kicks (strength exercise), 66
dopamine, 16–18, 23
Down Dog One Leg (yoga exercise),
    88
Down Dog (yoga exercise), 86
drinks: sample 14-day plan for,
    46–48

driving: cell phones/texting while, 92
dry cleaning: health tips about, 91

eating disorders
    biology of movement and, 14
    classic signs of, 42–43
    strategies for weight loss and,
        39–43
eating disorders not otherwise
        specified (EDNOS), 41–42
eating rituals, 43
eating too little. *See* deprivation diets
emergency foods, 32–33
emotions: biology of, 15–21
endorphins, 13
energy
    biology of fat and, 6, 7
    biology of hunger and, 7, 8, 9
    biology of movement and, 12, 13,
        14, 15
energy drinks, 37–38
environment
    eating disorders and, 42
    importance of, 24
    influence on biology of, 23–24
    inpact on behavior of, 23–24
    weight management and, 2, 21
exercise
beginner's guidelines for, 37–39
    benefits of, 13
    binge/excessive, 38, 43
    biology of movement and, 11–15
    cardiovascular, 37, 92
    as component of weight
        management plan, 45, 64–90
    eating disorders and, 41, 42, 43
    fantastic four, 35–37
    for flexibility, 37
    health tips about, 92
    hydration during, 37–38
    metabolism and, 13
    reasons for weight gain and, 22
    sample 14-day plan for, 46–48
    strategies for weight loss and,
        34–39
    and walking, 35

    See also band workout; strength
        training/workout; *specific
        exercise*
Extended Cat Stretch (yoga exercise),
    84

failure: planning for, 39
fantastic four, 35–37
fast food, 22, 31
fasting, 26–27
fat
    biology and, 5–24
    fretting about, 30–31
    kinds of, 6
    risk factors for too much, 5
    strategies for weight loss and,
        30–31
    See also type of fat
fats
    automating eating and, 27–28
    biology of hunger and, 7, 8
    function of, 8
    and no-fat diet, 30
    reasons for weight gain and, 22
    sources of, 7, 25
    strategies for weight loss and, 25,
        26, 27–28, 30
fiber
    biology of hunger and, 8
    sources of, 25, 26
    strategies for weight loss and, 25,
        26, 28
fidgeting, 12
Figure Eight Warm-up (band
        exercise), 69–70
five food felons, 26, 91–92
flexibility
    exercise for, 37
    strategies for weight loss and, 37
flour
    as food felon, 26
    tips about, 93
food choices: biology of hunger and,
        7, 8–11
food felons, 11, 26, 92
formaldehyde, 91

INDEX

14-day meal plan, 45–48
fruit
    sample 14-day plan for, 46–48
    strategies for weight loss and, 32
    tips about, 93

gamma-aminobutyric acid (GABA),
    16–18
genetics, 12
ghrelin, 9–11
glucose, 8, 15
glycogen, 33–34
Goddess (yoga exercise), 83
Going to Jail (band exercise), 74
good-for-YOU-foods group, 27–28
grocery shopping, 24
Ground to Sky (strength exercise),
    64–65

habits: components of weight
    management plans and, 45
Half Boat (yoga exercise), 89
Half Butterfly (yoga exercise), 90
Half Frog Pose (yoga exercise), 87
Hamstring Hang (strength exercise), 65
happiness: biology of fat and, 7
Harper, Joel, 69
healthful/unhealthful ingredients:
    strategies for weight loss and,
    25–26
heart
    biology of fat and, 7
    biology of movement and, 13,
    14–15
helmets: tips about, 93
high-fructose corn syrup (HFCS),
    10–11, 22, 26
hormones: strategies for weight loss
    and, 33
Horse (yoga exercise), 82
hunger
    biology of, 7–11
    confusing thirst and, 33
    denial of, 43
    strategies for weight loss and, 33
hypothalamus, 9

ingredients: healthful/unhealthful,
    25–26
insulin, 6, 17
Internet: health tips about, 93
Invisible Chair (strength exercise), 68

*The Journal of the American Medical
    Association,* 27
JP's Mac and Cheese
    recipe for, 56
    sample 14-day meal plan and, 48

Ladybug (yoga exercise), 81
Lateral Circle (band exercise), 71
Lateral Hold (band exercise), 72
Lateral Pull-Down (band exercise), 72
Lateral Raise (band exercise), 71
leptin, 9–11
Lifestyle 180 Banana Steel-Cut
    Oatmeal with Cinnamon
    (recipe), 51–52
Lifestyle 180 Berry-Banana Smoothie
    recipe for, 50
    sample 14-day meal plan and,
    46, 48
Lifestyle 180 Chia Sausage or
    Meatballs (recipe), 61–62
Lifestyle 180 Choose Your Fruit
    Pancakes (recipe), 52–53
Lion (yoga exercise), 84–85
Little Boat Pose (yoga exercise), 88
Little Boat Twist (yoga exercise),
    88–89
liver: biology of fat and, 5–6
lunch: sample meal plans for, 46–48

meal plans, 45–48
Mediterranean diet: strategies for
    weight loss and, 26, 27, 38
memory, 13
mental set: as component of weight
    management plan, 45
mentors, 93
metabolism
    biology and, 6, 7, 8, 11–15
    definition of, 11–12

exercise and, 13
   genetics and, 12
   hypothalamus and, 9
mirror neurons, 22
mood
   biology and, 7, 11, 13, 16, 17
   eating disorders and, 42, 43
   reasons for weight gain and, 22
movement: biology of, 11–15
multivitamins, 92
muscles
   biology of movement and, 13–14, 15
   core, 36
   flexibility exercise and, 37
   See also strength training/workout

Neck Stretch (band exercise), 71
nitric oxide, 16–18, 20, 79
noise: health tips about, 92
norepinephrine, 16–18

oats: strategies for weight loss and, 32
obesity
   as infectious disease, 29
   psychological issues concerned with, 18–19
   strategies for weight loss and, 29
omega-3 fatty acids, 25, 26, 28, 30, 31, 92
omega-9 fats, 28
omental fat, 6
omentum, 5–6
One-Foot Hop (strength exercise), 68
oxytocin, 19–20

Palms Out (band exercise), 73
passion: importance of, 92
Penguin (band exercise), 74–75
The Perfect Storm (movie), 23
perfection, 40
personal care products: health tips about, 91
pick and stick strategy, 28–29
Pineapple-Banana Protein Blaster (recipe), 51

plan/planning
   contingency, 39
   for failure, 39
   strategies for weight loss and, 27–28, 31–33
   See also plan, weight management
plan, weight management
   components of, 45
   exercise/workouts as component of, 45, 64–90
   recipes for, 49–64
   sample 14-day meal plan, 45–48
   strategies for weight loss and, 27–28, 31–33
portion size. *See* quantity of food
processed food, 10, 22, 93
protein
   automating eating and, 28
   biology of hunger and, 7, 8
   biology of movement and, 12
   function of, 7, 8
   sources of, 7, 25, 26
   strategies for weight loss and, 25, 26, 28
purging: eating disorders and, 41, 43

Quad Bend (strength exercise), 66–67
quality of food, 8–11
quantity of food, 7, 8–11

RB's Vegetarian Chili
   recipe for, 57–58
   sample 14-day meal plan and, 47
recipe(s)
   Black Bean Soup, 53–54
   burgers, 50
   Cinnamon Apple Sauté à la Mode, 63
   JP's Mac and Cheese, 56
   Lifestyle 180 Banana Steel-Cut Oatmeal with Cinnamon, 51–52
   Lifestyle 180 Berry-Banana Smoothie, 50
   Lifestyle 180 Chia Sausage or Meatballs, 61–62

recipe(s) (*continued*)
Lifestyle 180 Choose Your Fruit Pancakes, 52–53
Pineapple-Banana Protein Blaster, 51
RB's Vegetarian Chili, 57–58
salad, 49
sample, 49–64
sandwich, 49
Sesame Cucumber Salad, 54
Sliced Peaches with Raspberries, Blueberries, and Chocolate Chips, 63–64
smoothies, 49
snacks, 49–50
Spicy, Crunchy Garlic Broccoli and Cauliflower, 55
Stuffed Whole Wheat Pizza, 58–59
Tofu or Turkey Dogs with Sauerkraut, 60
Tomato-Avocado Salsamole, 62
Turkey Tortilla Wraps with Red Baked Potato, 59–60
resistance exercise, 92
Roll and Massage Back (yoga exercise), 88

salad
recipes for, 49
sample 14-day meal plan and, 46–48
salt: reasons for weight gain and, 22
sample 14-day plan. *See* plan, weight management
sandwiches: recipes for, 49
saturated fats, 26, 91–92
seat belts, 93
sedentary lifestyle, 22
self-esteem, 7, 18–20
self-image, 40, 42
serotonin, 11, 16–18
Sesame Cucumber Salad (recipe), 54
sex: health tips about, 93
Shoulder Height (band exercise), 73
Side Curl (band exercise), 74

Side Triceps Extension (band exercise), 73
skipping meals, 12. *See also* deprivation diet
sleep, 12, 13, 92
Sliced Peaches with Raspberries, Blueberries, and Chocolate Chips (recipe), 63–64
smoothies: recipes for, 49
snacks
recipes for, 49–50
sample meal plans for, 46–48
socialization: strategies for weight loss and, 29
soft drinks, 33
soups: strategies for weight loss and, 32
Spicy, Crunchy Garlic Broccoli and Cauliflower (recipe), 55
Spinal Twist (band exercise), 77
Squat (band exercise), 75
Standing Chest Press (band exercise), 70
Standing Chest Pull (band exercise), 70
Standing Leaning Stretch (yoga exercise), 80
Standing Twist (yoga exercise), 80
starvation. *See* deprivation diet; fasting
Stork (yoga exercise), 82
strategies for weight loss, 25–43
beginner guidelines for, 37–39
calorie counting and, 27
eating disorders and, 39–43
exercise and, 34–39
fat and, 30–31
guidelines for, 37–39
healthful/unhealthful ingredients and, 25–26
management plan for, 27–28
plan for failure and, 39
planning your meals and, 31–33
socialization and, 29
sticking to your plan and, 28–29
thirst and, 33

undereating and, 26–27
weight range and, 33–34
strength training/workout
  Air Angels, 65–66
  Armcopter, 65
  Back Bend, 67
  Break Dancing, 67–68
  Crisscross, 64
  Donkey Kicks, 66
  fantastic four and, 35, 36
  Ground to Sky, 64–65
  Hamstring Hang, 65
  Invisible Chair, 68
  One-Foot Hop, 68
  Quad Bend, 66–67
  strategies for weight loss and, 35, 36
  Triceps Push-ups, 66
  Zigzag, 67
stress
  biology of emotions and, 16
  eating disorders and, 40, 42
  health tips about, 92
  reasons for weight gain and, 22
Stuffed Whole Wheat Pizza
  recipe for, 58–59
  sample 14-day meal plan and, 46, 48
subcutaneous fat, 6
sugars
  biology and, 8, 11, 14–15, 17
  as food felon, 26, 92
  function of, 8
  health tips about, 92
  reasons for weight gain and, 22
  strategies for weight loss and, 32
syrup: as food felon, 26, 92

teeth: health tips about, 92
texting: health tips about, 92, 93
thirst
  confusing hunger and, 33
  strategies for weight loss and, 33, 37–38
Thread the Needle (band exercise), 76
Thread the Needle (yoga exercise), 84

Tightrope (yoga exercise), 81
tips, health, 91–93
tobacco, 91
Tofu or Turkey Dogs with Sauerkraut
  recipe for, 60
  sample 14-day meal plan and, 46
Tomato-Avocado Salsamole
  recipe for, 62
  sample 14-day meal plan and, 47
toxins: health tips about, 91
trans fats, 26, 91–92
Tree (yoga exercise), 81–82
Triangle (yoga exercise), 83
Triceps Push-ups (strength exercise), 66
triglycerides, 5–6
Turkey Tortilla Wraps with Red Baked Potato
  recipe for, 59–60
  sample 14-day meal plan and, 47

undereating
  eating disorders and, 43
  strategies for weight loss and, 26–27
unhealthful foods (food felons), 11, 26, 92
unsaturated fats, 25

vaccinations, 92
vegetables
  health tips about, 92, 93
  sample 14-day plan for, 46–48
  strategies for weight loss and, 32, 39

waist-to-height ratio, 92
walking, 34, 35, 38, 39, 46, 91
warm-up exercises, 69–70
weight
  range for, 33–34
  teen angst about, 1–2
  tips about managing, 91–93
weight gain: reasons for, 21–23
weight loss
  band workout and, 69–77

INDEX

weight loss (*continued*)
    drugs for, 16
    healthful/unhealthful ingredients
      and, 25–26
    sample 14-day meal plan for,
      45–48
    sample recipes for, 49–64
    strategies for, 25–43
    strength training/workout and,
      36, 64–68
    yoga and, 78–90
whole grains: as food felon, 26, 92
workouts. *See* exercise; *specific exercise*
    or type of exercise
Wrist Extensions (yoga exercise), 85

X (yoga exercise), 80–81

Yoga Lunges (yoga exercise), 86
Yoga workout, 78–90
    benefits of, 78–79
    Butterfly, 89
    Camel, 85
    Cat Back/Cow, 83–84
    Cobra, 86–87
    Corpse, 90
    Diagonal Reach, 87

Down Dog, 86
Down Dog One Leg, 88
Extended Cat Stretch, 84
Goddess, 83
guidelines for, 79–80
Half Boat, 89
Half Butterfly, 90
Half Frog Pose, 87
Horse, 82
Ladybug, 81
Lion, 84–85
Little Boat Pose, 88
Little Boat Twist, 88–89
Roll and Massage Back, 88
Standing Leaning Stretch, 80
Standing Twist, 80
Stork, 82
Thread the Needle exercise, 84
Tightrope, 81
Tree, 81–82
Triangle, 83
Wrist Extensions, 85
X, 80–81
Yoga Lunges, 86

Zigzag (strength exercise), 67
zits: health tips about, 93

ABOUT THE AUTHORS

MICHAEL F. ROIZEN, MD, is a *New York Times* number one bestselling author and cofounder and originator of the very popular RealAge website. He is chief wellness officer and chair of the Wellness Institute of the Cleveland Clinic and the chief medical consultant of *The Dr. Oz Show.*

MEHMET C. OZ, MD, is also a *New York Times* number one bestselling author and three-time Emmy Award–winning host of *The Dr. Oz Show.* He is professor and vice chairman of surgery at New York Presbyterian-Columbia University Medical Center and the director of the Heart Institute.

ELLEN ROME, MD, MPH, is head of adolescent medicine at the Cleveland Clinic Children's Hospital. She is a board-certified pediatrician who is among the first in the country to also be board-certified in adolescent medicine. Dr. Rome received her undergraduate degree from Yale University, her medical degree from Case Western Reserve University's School of Medicine, and her master's in public health from Harvard's School of Public Health.